Helping Your
ELDERLY
PATIENTS
A guide for
Nursing Assistants

JUDITH M. CONAHAN, MSN

THE TIRESIAS PRESS, INC., NEW YORK CITY

Library of Congress
Catalog Card Number: 75-40507
International Standard
Book Number: 0-913292-29-X

Printed in U.S.A.

Current printing (last digit): 10 9 8 7 6 5 4 3 2

To Nellie

Drawings by Peter Dixon. Photographs by Peter Calkins.

ABOUT THE AUTHOR

JUDITH M. CONAHAN received her diploma in
nursing from the Henry Ford Hospital School of
Nursing in Detroit, her BS from Wayne State
University, and her MS in Nursing from Boston
University, where she specialized in community
health nursing and gerontology.

Helping Your Elderly Patients evolved from a
series of workshops on the psychosocial care of
the elderly that Mrs. Conahan planned and
implemented for nursing assistants from long-term
care facilities. The workshops were sponsored by
the Massachusetts Department of Public Health.
The nursing assistants' interest in the material, and
their desire to have it in written form for future
reference, gave the author the impetus to write this
book, which is designed to complement the text on
physical skills customarily studied by nursing
assistants. Mrs. Conahan now teaches nursing
home personnel at the New England Rehabilitation
Hospital in Woburn, Massachusetts.

Preface

The purpose of this book is to help nursing assistants understand the important role they assume when caring for older persons, and to increase their awareness of, and sensitivity to, the needs of their elderly patients.

Nursing assistants are responsible for a large part of the care given to residents of long-term care facilities. They are in close contact with them for long periods of time, and are most available to provide the comfort and caring residents need. Yet, traditionally, their training has not included emotional or psychosocial aspects of care.

The material in this book evolved from my work in planning and giving workshops for nursing assistants working in long-term care facilities throughout Massachusetts. The workshops focused on the psychosocial aspects of care for the elderly. The nursing assistants who attended the workshops enjoyed the opportunity to talk about their feelings and their work. Many of them wished they could obtain more information in writing.

This book is meant to be read by nursing assistants. It assumes some previous introduction to the long-term care setting. In-service instructors may find it of use during the initial training period, along with a book on physical skills. Continuing education instructors may similarly find it useful.

The discussion questions at the end of most chapters will help nursing assistants relate the information in each chapter to their own settings and patients. The case studies and role plays in Chapters Eight and Nine are designed to stimulate discussion of some common problems. The bibliographies and list of audiovisual aids at the end of the book are included so that instructors and nursing assistants can have readily available a comprehensive list of educational materials for further study.

This book would not have been written without the help and interest of many people.   I am particularly grateful to Marian Spencer, Associate Professor of Nursing at Boston University, who began the project and has supported me with her knowledge, experience, and encouragement. A special thank you goes to my family.

Judith M. Conahan

Contents

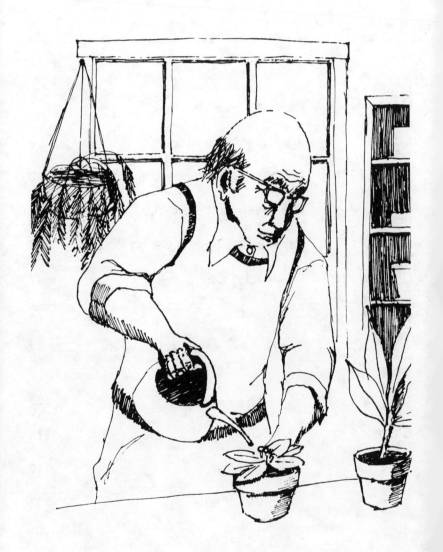

1

Introduction

The human life span has changed little if at all throughout the history of man. The fittest of us rarely live longer than about 105 years. But, due to better living conditions, food, and health care, *more* people are living longer. In fact, one in every ten Americans (20.1 million people) is 65 years of age or older. In 1900 only one in every 25 Americans was over 65. The percentage of older people in the American population has doubled since 1900.[1]

This is an important figure to those in the health field who work with the elderly. As people get older, the chance that they will become permanently ill and dependent increases. As of 1972, at least one out of every 20 older Americans (about one million in all) lived in institutions of one type or another. Even though most elderly people live in family settings, physical or emotional changes may eventually require specialized nursing care in institutions.

Although many older people prefer to live alone, others enter institutions when they no longer have friends or relatives to help them. With increasing age more people become more alone. Many more women are alone than men because in the elderly population there are about 138 women to every 100 men. Also, many more women are widowed. Most older men are married and living with their wives.

Some older people enter institutions because they cannot afford to support and feed themselves. They need to pay more for health care and have less to pay other bills with. About one in every seven older persons works outside of the home. Others depend solely on Social Security, pensions (if they have them), and old age assistance from the government. In 1971, 22 percent (4.3 million) of all older people in the United States lived below the poverty level.

Many of these people worked very hard all their lives. They grew up around the turn of the century when most people believed that success was attained by hard work and self-sacrifice. Being dependent and accepting any form of charity, even a government subsidy, was viewed as a sign of failure. Because of these beliefs, many older people today do not seek assistance when they need it. And when they must enter an institution, they may feel ashamed.

Unless more community and home health services are provided, there will be more and more elderly people in nursing homes in the future. This will increase the need for people who have been especially educated to understand the problems and needs of this group of people.

The care of chronically ill older people in long-term care facilities (nursing homes) calls for treatment just as specialized as that given to acutely ill people in hospitals. In long-term care, however, the goal is different. It is not necessarily to "get the patients better" or to "cure" them, but to help them function as well as possible.

Those who care for the elderly are concerned with the *quality* of their patients' lives. Many times nothing can be done to extend the number of years that a person will live, but much can be done to make the present a time when he can be proud of himself, care about himself, and look forward to each day.

Aging is a universal process that can be denied, but that cannot be escaped. Those who work in long-term care facilities with many patients and little time sometimes lose sight of the person within the aged body. The person within, no matter how old, has the same needs and desires as everyone else. Everyone wants to feel wanted, loved, and useful.

In the following chapters, it is hoped that you will gain a better understanding of who the aged are and how you, as a member of a nursing team, can help them help themselves. It is important that you realize how much your presence, appearance, and actions can affect the functioning of your elderly patients. By gaining a new knowledge and awareness about the aged and aging, your job will be more satisfying to you, and you will be more helpful to your patients.

REFERENCE:

[1] All statistics in this chapter were taken from: U.S. Department of Health, Education, and Welfare, Office of Human Development, Administration on Aging, "New Facts about Older Americans" (Washington D.C. 20402: Superintendent of Documents, U.S. Government Printing Office, DHEW Publication N. [SRS] 73-20006, June 1973).

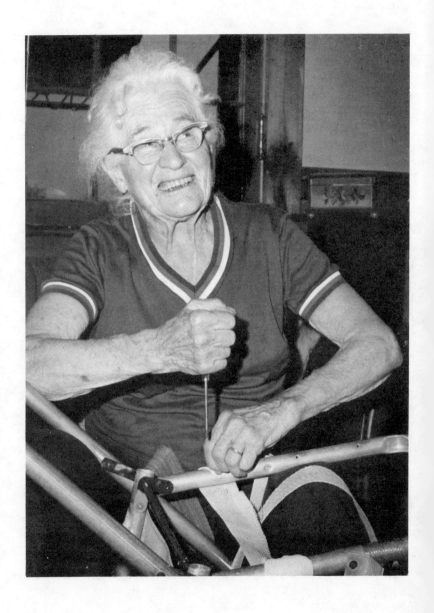

2

A Closer Look at the Aging Process

According to one dictionary definition, human aging is a process of deterioration that results in bodily changes which cannot be reversed. People are often considered elderly or aged when they reach the age of 65, the age at which most people retire from their work. But a person's chronological age (the number of years he has lived) does not necessarily indicate his physical or mental age. The saying, "you're as old as you feel," is true.

Aging can also be defined as the process of growing older. People begin growing and aging at birth, maybe even at conception. Old age is a continuation of this process, a time of maturing and ripening, the last stage of growth in the life cycle. The physical signs of aging (gray hair, wrinkles, stooped posture) may give the impression of deterioration. But physical signs do not necessarily reflect how well the body is functioning nor the state of the mind.

STAGES OF DEVELOPMENT

Throughout our lives, we have to deal with new problems and tasks. These problems and tasks are generally similar for all of us, depending upon where we are in the life cycle.

The stages of development that make up the life cycle are: Early Childhood (1-5 years), Childhood and Adolescence (5-21), Adulthood (21-45), Middle Years (45-65), Later Maturity (65-75), and Old Age (75 on).[1]

During Adulthood the tasks usually involve a career or job, marriage, and a family. This is a time for obtaining things— possessions, relationships, position, status, and so on. It is a time of achievement.

The Middle Years are a time of stabilization. There is a reevaluation of one's life and life style in the light of an aging body, children leaving home, and future retirement. People begin to look for new ways to use their time and begin to plan for old age.

During Later Maturity and Old Age, people experience many losses. They may begin to prepare for the final loss, their own death. This preparation may be obvious, as when people give away their possessions or talk about their coming death, or it may occur only as fleeting thoughts about the deaths of others or of one's self. Those who have become grandparents (and often those who have not) look for some connection to other generations. People in these stages of life tend to become less afraid than before of showing their individuality. At the same time, they begin to examine the significance of their lives.

COPING WITH CHANGES AND LOSSES

This generation of elderly has seen many changes in its lifetime, more than any other generation before it. In the past 50 years, the way people live has changed tremendously because of technological developments. Many of these developments have made the skills of older people outdated. In addition, changes in the moral attitudes of society seem to negate the religious and other beliefs that these people relied on to direct their lives.

One of the major tasks of older people is learning to cope with many losses and changes over a relatively short period of time. And they have to do this at a time in their lives when they have less energy with which to cope.

Some of these losses and changes include:

Biological Changes

- Decreased ability to work due to weakening muscles, less energy, and changes in the circulatory and respiratory systems.

- Decreased ability to see, smell, taste, and hear.

- Increased risk of getting heart disease, diabetes, cancer, and stroke.

- Thinning of the bones and changes in the joints which limit range of motion.

- A slowing down of the nervous system that results in slower responses. Walking and other coordinated movements now require forethought and care.

- Decreased fine coordinated movements *when hurried.*

Emotional and Psychological Changes

● Having to accommodate to a new self-image as the body changes.

● Decreased ability to remember recent events.

● Having to face the nearness of death and dying.

Social Changes

● Reduced income; changed living standards; possible loss of home.

● Retirement from work; more leisure time; loss of purpose.

● Loss of status in the community and family.

● Loss of many significant people and possessions in life.

● Isolation.

● Possible institutionalization or relocation.

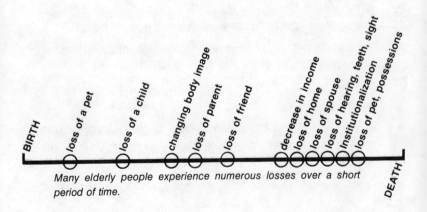

Many elderly people experience numerous losses over a short period of time.

Any personal loss, as of a friend, relative, or prized possession, can seriously affect a person's functioning. He may be
slowed down mentally and physically for weeks and even
months after such a loss. This may interfere with performing the
normal activities of daily living. As people grow older, they
experience more and more losses closer and closer together,
without time for recovery. Placement in a nursing home may be
seen by an elder as the final loss, and he may act confused and
disoriented. Under the circumstances, this is justified behavior.
A younger person would probably act the same way in the same
situation.

STEREOTYPING THE ELDERLY

Not only do older people have to endure loss and disap-
pointment, but they must live in a society which, on the whole, is
prejudiced against them. In the United States, there are many
negative attitudes toward aging. This stereotyping or categoriz-
ing of people because they are old is called "agism."[2] It is
similar to sexism and racism in that people with *some* similar
characteristics are grouped together and thought to have *other*
similar characteristics. Some of these common stereotypes
are:

"Older people are senile or in their second childhood."

The term *senility* refers to deterioration, usually mental.
Calling a person senile is a convenient way of labeling him
as someone for whom nothing more can be done. Too

often, when we can't understand a patient's behavior, we feel helpless about it, and say, "But he's senile," which seems to explain the situation. When the doctor talks about the senile patient, he is referring to someone with the diagnosis of chronic organic brain syndrome (irreversible brain damage). The word senile is a "wastebasket" term that should be eliminated from our vocabulary. Instead, we should be describing patients' behaviors and trying to find reasons for them.

"Older people look alike."

Sometimes we let the more obvious signs of old age interfere with seeing older people as individuals. The less contact we have with this age group the more likely we are to make this mistake. Not only must we consider the differences in the physical characteristics and personalities of people, but we must also consider the differences in their ages. A 65-year-old person and an 85-year-old person are both "older Americans." But the 85-year-old person was born 20 years earlier and would have been old enough to be the parent of the 65-year-old person!

"Older people are not productive citizens. They can no longer produce on the job, or be creative."

Retirement is mandatory for most jobs, but there are many famous aged musicians, scientists, and painters, as well as many other old people who work regularly, both full and part time.

"Older people think and act alike, resist change, and cannot make decisions."

Personality traits learned throughout life produce individual ways of being old. Some older people cannot make decisions and cannot change. They couldn't when they were 25 years old either. Others can and have always been able to.

"Older people 'reap what they sow,' live in serenity, and enjoy the 'fruits of their labor.'"

Many people who have labored and saved their money cannot support themselves today. Millions of the aged live in extreme poverty.

SUCCESSFUL AGING

Today, because of medical and technological advances, more people live longer. However, because they live in a society which highly values youth, independence, and the idea of obsolescence (replacing that which is worn or broken), the later years can be difficult ones. Despite this, many people have a satisfying, successful old age.

Each person adapts to aging in his own way. Some view with insight the years they have lived. They try to overcome their weaknesses and take advantage of their strengths. Others take advantage of their weaknesses and use them as excuses for their declining abilities. Some enjoy their role of dependence, feeling that they have done their share of work and deserve to rest. Others blame the rest of the world (including the people who care for them) for their difficulties. All of these people have adapted to aging, some more successfully than others.

Many factors may contribute to happiness or success in old age. These may include having money, good health, education, family support, and a good diet. They may include having opportunities for learning, for expressing oneself creatively, or for being useful and productive. Maybe the ability and desire to remain mentally and physically active and involved in life brings happiness. Or maybe it is an attitude or state of mind that helps some people age successfully.

An important factor in successful aging is a person's ability to cope with and adapt to change. How one copes with change reflects behavior patterns that were learned in childhood. Parents should teach children a positive approach to aging by their own example. Often children get to know very few older people, or they see them only in television commercials for sleeping pills, denture pastes, or laxatives.

Sharon Curtin aptly observed a parent's effect on her child's learning.[3] The child asked her mother why her grandmother had to use a special wooden bowl when she ate. The mother replied that the grandmother was so old and feeble that she kept dropping and breaking the china dishes. After thinking a minute, the daughter said that the wooden bowl should be saved so that her mother could also use it when she got old.

We cannot spend a lifetime denying our own aging. We must prepare for it.

SUMMARY

In order to understand elderly people, you must examine your own feelings toward aging and the aged. It is difficult to care for an older person and deny aging at the same time. This chapter has given you some information about the aging process. Now you must look and listen more closely to the elderly around you.

REFERENCES

[1]Louis Lowy, *Training Manual for Human Service Technicians. Working with Older Persons, Part II Trainees* (Boston: United Community Services of Metropolitan Boston, 1968), pp. 21-25.

[2]Robert N. Butler, and Myrna I. Lewis, *Aging and Mental Health* (St. Louis: The C.V. Mosby Company, 1973), p. ix.

[3]Sharon Curtin, *Nobody Ever Died of Old Age* (Boston: Little Brown and Company, 1972), pp. 196-7.

DISCUSSION QUESTIONS

1. Choose a patient from your facility. How does he or she compare with the facts given in this chapter about elderly people?

2. Discuss the differences in the life styles of 65- and 85-year-old people when they were children.

3. What is successful aging? Think of one of your patients who seems to have aged successfully. What characteristics does this patient have that probably contributed to this success?

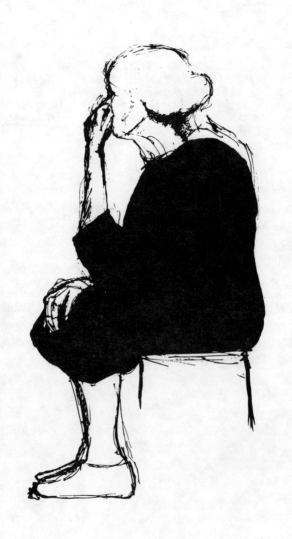

3

The Needs of the Elderly

All human beings, including the elderly, have the same basic needs. These needs are: 1) the physical needs—food and fluids, clothing, shelter, elimination, activity, rest, and, possibly, sexual expression, 2) the need for safety and security, 3) the need to love and belong, 4) the need for self-esteem and self-respect, and 5) the need for self-realization.

These basic needs are progressive. This means that the physical needs are the most basic and that the need for self-realization is the least basic. When people are uncomfortable, they are concerned about fulfilling their most basic needs first.[1] The starving person is more concerned about how to get food than about what other people think of him. The nursing home resident who is afraid of losing her purse will be more concerned about watching and holding it than about concentrating on her cards in a Bingo game. The patient who is worried about being incontinent will be more concerned about not wetting himself than about dressing up to impress his family when they come for a visit.

Older people want to continue to meet their needs by themselves, but it may be hard for them to do this. Those in

23

nursing homes need special help to find ways to meet their needs that will help them stay as independent as possible. Nursing assistants should look for ways to help patients do this. When you observe that a patient's needs are not being met, talk with both the patient and your supervisor about it. Then you and the rest of the nursing team should search for ways to meet the patient's needs.

A discussion of these needs and how older people must adapt to meet them follows.

BASIC PHYSICAL NEEDS

Food and Fluids

Older people have the same nutritional needs for fats, protein, and carbohydrates as younger people, except that they need fewer calories. However, they may not get adequate nutrition for many reasons.

As a person ages, movement of food along his digestive tract may be slowed. There may be a decrease in the stomach and bowel secretions that help digest the food. The stomach may not be able to hold as much food and fluid as it once did. Many older people may prefer to eat several small meals and a bedtime snack rather than three large meals. When possible, this should be encouraged.

Older people may not be able to chew as well as when they were younger. They may need false teeth or specially prepared food. Most people dislike minced and pureed foods and would prefer to have well-fitted false teeth. Some, however, can barely chew with or without teeth due to arthritic changes in the jaw.

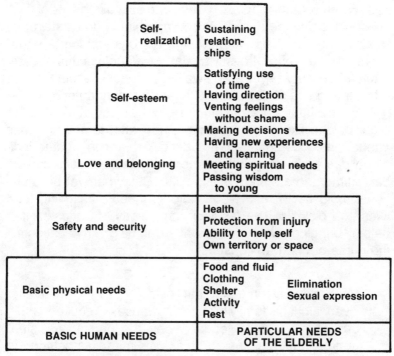

BASIC HUMAN NEEDS	PARTICULAR NEEDS OF THE ELDERLY
Self-realization	Sustaining relationships
Self-esteem	Satisfying use of time Having direction Venting feelings without shame Making decisions
Love and belonging	Having new experiences and learning Meeting spiritual needs Passing wisdom to young
Safety and security	Health Protection from injury Ability to help self Own territory or space
Basic physical needs	Food and fluid Clothing Shelter Elimination Activity Sexual expression Rest

A chart of basic human needs

Some elders lose their appetite because their senses of smell and taste have declined. For the same reason, many older people like strongly flavored food. Some elders have a bad taste in their mouths and need mouth care before every meal. Some will not eat because they cannot move well enough to feed themselves, or because they are tired, unhappy, or lonely. Since most of them have eaten with others in the past, this should be encouraged whenever possible.

When someone needs your help to eat, take plenty of time. Sit down facing the patient. Encourage him to do whatever he possibly can to assist you, even if it is only holding a straw. Never feed anyone who is lying flat in bed unless this is absolutely necessary. With age, swallowing often becomes more difficult and could result in choking and regurgitation.

Eating habits are developed over a lifetime. What each older person likes, how he eats it, and what it means to him cannot easily be changed. It is difficult to accommodate individual desires in an institution where all meals are served at the same time and are pretty much alike. But, wherever possible, you should try to meet your patients' needs, including food likes and dislikes. The families and friends of patients often help by bringing favorite foods which can be given to patients if the nurse or dietitian consents.

Mr. Smith was on a diet that restricted his protein intake. Every night his family brought him pieces of cooked rabbit, one of his favorite foods. When the nursing assistant realized that, because of this, Mr. Smith was getting too much protein, she talked to the nurse about it. Arrangements were made with the dietitian whereby the patient would be allowed to substitute the rabbit for the meat in his evening meals.

Getting residents involved in planning and preparing a monthly meal might be one way of accommodating individual likes. Some homes occasionally plan meals with a theme. The theme might be a specific nationality, such as Italian, Greek, German, etc., or a holiday. A nursing assistant might suggest such an idea and become involved in planning it.

Dehydration caused by too limited a fluid intake is a problem with many older people, especially those in nursing home. Some drink less because fluids are not made easily available to them. Nursing assistants should be sure that fluids *are* available at all times. Some elders drink less because they are afraid of involuntarily dribbling urine or of having to get up at night to go to the bathroom. Actually, by not drinking they are making the problem worse. Drinking sufficient fluids helps increase the tone and holding capacity of the bladder and also prevents the formation of stones.

Clothing

People living in nursing homes need to be encouraged to dress in their own clothing every day. They also need opportunities, such as those provided by social activities, outings, or dinners, to get specially "dressed up." Clothes should be clean and bright and should be replaced at regular intervals. Every resident should have a choice of "what to wear today."

Clothing for the elderly needs to be designed for the bodily changes that occur with increasing age. These changes may include a shortening in height, a curving out of the back, a backward tilt of the head, a smaller chest, narrower shoulders, more fat in the hips and abdomen and less fat in the arms and legs, and a slight bending of the hips and knees. Clothing should be lightweight and easy to take off and put on. Clothing should not restrict the patient's circulation or breathing, and should not be irritating to the skin.

Shelter

While older patients or residents are in a nursing home, it is their home. Is it possible to make the institution more homelike? What makes your own home comfortable? The colors of the walls, furniture, and curtains, the warmth of people who know and accept you, or being surrounded by familiar objects and possessions—these are some of the things that contribute to a home-like atmosphere.

Mrs. Vandrorn resided in a nursing home for the last few years of her life. One day she was found sitting on her bed with an apron on. When asked why, she said, "Because it feels so good." This woman, who had spent most of her adult life in her own house, could find no comfortable place in her present "home." People need to continue some of their life activities if possible. If a former housewife cannot cook or bake, maybe she could help plan menus or set the table or trays.

Elimination

Bowel and bladder incontinence (passing of stool or urine at inappropriate times) is a serious problem among the elderly. Many enter nursing homes because of it.

Bladder Incontinence.   With age, the urinary bladder and its opening weaken. The nerves that carry messages to tell people when they have to urinate also weaken. As a result, older people have to urinate more frequently. They may have to get up to go to the bathroom during the night. Sometimes they may involuntarily dribble urine.

Because of these bodily changes, any additional stress, such as moving to a nursing home, losing a loved one, or being confined to bed, may result in incontinence. Disease that causes brain damage or infection in the bladder or in other parts of the body may do the same thing. An enlarged prostate gland frequently causes incontinence in the older male.

No matter what the cause of incontinence, it is embarrassing for those who experience it. Many incontinent people prefer to stay in their rooms. Gradually, they lose interest in the people around them.

If your patient appears to be incontinent, observe how much contact he or she has with other people during the day. Talk with the patient frequently. Encourage him to wear his own clothing. One incontinent resident never wet himself when he wore his own clothing.

Observe how often the incontinent person urinates. What times during the day and night must he go to the bathroom or does he wet himself? Some residents might not be incontinent if they were reminded at regular intervals (after meals, on awakening, before bed, before physical activity) to go to the bathroom.

Observe the amount of liquid the incontinent person drinks during the day. Many older people drink very few fluids. They believe that by drinking less they will dribble less. In time, however, drinking small amounts of fluids may make incontinence worse! The bladder needs to fill to its normal capacity. Otherwise, it will shrink so that it holds less urine and the patient will have to urinate more often.

Observe the position of the incontinent patient when he is urinating. It is difficult to completely empty the bladder when one is lying on a bedpan. Urine that is left in the bladder when it is not completely emptied stagnates. This causes infection and stones, which can increase incontinence. If at all possible, people should sit up to urinate.

Observe how much assistance your incontinent patient needs to urinate, and promptly answer his calls. If the bladder is overfull for any length of time, it becomes stretched. Also, the urge to urinate may become less strong. Urine dribbles out without the person being aware of it.

Try to understand what the patient is feeling. If he is tense, hurt, or angry, the incontinence may get worse. A special effort must be made to treat the patient with respect. He should not be scolded like a child who has wet his pants, but should be treated as an adult who is having a problem and needs assistance.

Those who are incontinent only at night may need to have their fluid intake reduced in the evening. They should be awakened at night to go to the bathroom, or be put on a bedpan, commode, or urinal. This is the only circumstance under which fluids should be restricted, unless a specific order has been given.

Many incontinent people could benefit from a bladder control program. This can include those who have indwelling catheters. When a patient is placed on a bladder training program, it means that he is given measured amounts of fluids regularly throughout the day, and that he is placed on a commode or in the bathroom to empty his bladder at specific times throughout the day and night. These programs are planned and directed by the nursing staff. If your patients are involved in such programs, you will usually be responsible for providing them with fluids, reminding them to drink them at specific times, and recording how much they drink. You will also be responsible for helping them onto the commode or into the bathroom at specified times, and for measuring and recording the urine output. The success or failure of the training program may depend on how well you do these things.

Nursing assistants involved in bladder training programs should talk as much as possible with their patients. They should tell the patients why they should drink or go to the bathroom. They should help their patients stay meticulously clean and dry. They should report regularly to the nursing staff on how those on the training programs are feeling and how much they are urinating.

Some older people with severe degenerative changes may not benefit from a bladder training program and may need devices such as condoms, catheters, or specially padded underwear to help keep them dry. Frequent cleaning and drying of the perineal area is necessary to prevent skin breakdown. Special cleaning and care around the catheter should be done daily.

Constipation and Bowel Incontinence.   Control of the bowels is a problem of the elderly that can usually be helped. Many residents in nursing homes are constipated and worry about it. With age, the muscular movement of the bowel slows and weakens. In addition, other factors such as a change of diet, inactivity, medications, depression, and not enough fluids, slow down bowel functioning.

Nursing assistants can help patients by having fluids available for them, and by allowing them time to move their bowels. They should encourage patients to exercise moderately and to eat foods (unless they are on a special diet) with roughage, such as vegetables and fruit.

If a patient cannot get out of bed by himself he should be assisted onto a commode or toilet at the same time every day.

The natural sitting position is important to easy movement of the bowels. Those who are used to taking laxatives may need to take these at night so they can evacuate their bowels the next morning.

Bowel incontinence in the elderly is often caused by severe constipation or impaction. The person appears to have almost continuous liquid stool. But this liquid is seeping around a large hard piece of stool which cannot move out of the bowel. In fact, some people may be so constipated that they become confused. This onset of incontinence and confusion may be mistakenly interpreted as "senility," but it quickly disappears when the impaction is removed. Impaction may have to be removed by a suppository, digital manipulation, and/or enemas. All should be done by a specially trained person. When the impaction is removed, regular bowel habits can be re-established.

Nursing assistants should tell the nurse about any patient who has diarrhea or who has not had a bowel movement in more than three days. Such a patient may have a bowel impaction.

Activity

Our bodies need to move in order to function efficiently. Without movement our muscles become flabby and our minds become dull. Frequent position changes—lying, sitting, standing, and walking—are necessary for good circulation of the blood and an adequate supply of oxygen for the brain.

It is risky to leave an older person in bed or sitting in a chair for long periods of time during the day. Not only must he contend with the effects of aging, but also with the effects of inactivity. This means his heart may be overworked. The aged heart pumps out less blood than it once did. The aged lungs and rib cage are less elastic than they used to be. Not as much air is taken in and blown out of the lungs as when the patient was younger. Coughs are less forceful and secretions are harder to raise. The heart of anyone at any age who must lie flat or sit still most of the time has to work harder to pump enough blood to the rest of the body. The lungs cannot expand and contract as well in this position and they tend to collect mucus.

Almost every system of the body is affected in some way by reduced activity. Some other effects of inactivity include: 1) increased stiffening of the joints (contractures), 2) muscle weakness, 3) thrombophlebitis with the possibility that a clot may travel to the lung (pulmonary embolism), 4) bedsores (decubitus ulcers), 5) pneumonia, 6) kidney and bladder stones, 7) lighter and more brittle bones (osteoporosis), and 8) constipation. Thus, when an older person with an already slowed-down system is placed in a situation in which that system has to work harder, the chances for rapid breakdown increase.

Provision for activity of some sort should be made for every resident of the nursing home. People whom the doctor has ordered to remain in bed should be repositioned every two hours and have Range of Motion Exercises three or four times a day. Only nursing assistants who have been taught to do Range of Motion Exercises should do them or instruct patients how to do them.

Aside from those who have been ordered to remain in bed, everyone should be out of bed every day. Those who can only sit in chairs should be moved frequently. Instead of spending six consecutive hours in their chairs, they should spend three two-hour periods sitting, with rest periods in bed in between. While sitting, patients should be encouraged to shift their weight from side to side. If possible, the patient should join an exercise group. These are now becoming more common in nursing homes. In an exercise group, patients, either in chairs or standing, get into a circle with the staff and follow the movements of a leader. Sometimes the movements are easier and more fun to do when they are done to music. Those who can only move one side are encouraged to use their strong side to exercise the weak side. Patients who cannot move by themselves may be helped to go through the motions by a staff member.

You should always watch for what your patient can do by himself. You should encourage even the smallest movement, such as lifting a washcloth to the face. People benefit most, both physically and mentally, from movements they perform themselves.

Rest

Everyone needs rest. Older people tend to sleep fewer hours and less deeply than others. Some nursing home residents complain of not sleeping all night. Others are awakened frequently by aches and pains. Also, due to body changes, they may need to get up at night to urinate. With lessened activity, especially in long-term care facilities, they tend to nap during the day and to go to bed early in the evening. Consequently, they often can't sleep at night. Not only do they not sleep, they worry about not sleeping. They've been taught since childhood that it is necessary to get eight hours of sleep every night.

Older people need to be active during the day. However,

they need shorter periods of activity and more rest periods in between. Many do not have the energy for strenuous activity without frequent rest times to restore their energy. Nursing assistants should help them understand that they cannot be as active as when they were younger, and that they must heed signs of tiredness and plan frequent rest periods during the day.

Too often, doctors and nurses try to solve the problem of sleeplessness in older people by giving them sedatives. A nursing assistant's thoughtful care can induce a much better night's sleep than a pill. A backrub, a warm drink, a snack, or a short conversation may be all that is needed to make a resident feel relaxed enough to fall asleep. When you reassure him that he is safe and that someone will come if he calls, it is like another warm blanket.

Patients who are not confused at other times may become so at night. Adjusting to darkness is difficult for those who have lost some of their sight and hearing. Noises and shapes grow monstrously out of proportion. The curtains become ghosts and images of people out of the past. The sound of a dropped bedpan in the utility room is interpreted as a group of firemen. Quiet talking among nurses at the desk is heard in garbled snatches and may be interpreted by the patient as a plot against him. Siderails become prison bars.

Those patients who become confused at night should be well and frequently oriented to their rooms and the things in them. Orientation to siderails should be positive rather than negative. Tell the patient how the siderails keep him from falling rather than how they can prevent him from getting out of bed. Older people need a night light (15 watts), a call button within reach, and an understanding face and voice when they call.

Sexual Expression

A person is never too old for sexual expression. The elderly have sexual needs just as other adults do. Although the structure and function of the sex organs gradually change, people who have been sexually active during their lives can remain so well into the later years. In fact, because of the numerous losses of loved ones which increasing age brings, elderly people may have a great need for physical closeness and the warmth of another person.

Today's elderly people grew up at a time when sexual feelings were disapproved of and suppressed. Many of them learned to be ashamed of their sexual feelings and fantasies. Even those who do not feel this way may believe that sexual activity is somehow immoral or wrong now that they are old. Or they may think they can no longer experience pleasure from sex.

Many of the people who care for older people (including their children and grandchildren) agree that sexual desire is something elderly people should have outgrown. A patient who tries to touch nurses or other patients is immediately labeled a dirty old man or woman and is sometimes restrained or sedated.

Lots of people believe that their elders are just too infirm to engage in sexual intercourse. Yet such activity will not usually do any physical harm. In fact, the lack of sexual contact may cause some patients to become irritable and more disabled. Both the elderly and those who care for them should understand that, although the process is slower, sex can be as great a pleasure for the elderly as it is for younger people.

Nursing assistants who work in long-term care facilities must think about their own feelings regarding sexual expression in their elderly patients. Too often those who care for the elderly punish any behavior that seems to be of a sexual nature. It would be much better to find out why the person is doing what he is doing.

> For several days nursing assistants noticed that Miss Alcott, a prim and proper retired school teacher of 82, was scratching in her pubic area. The assistants were embarrassed and tried to keep her hands away from the area. They thought she was probably "getting senile." The patient was also embarrassed, but said she could not stop it. When the doctor visited her, he realized that she was having a drug reaction (itching was a symptom). He immediately stopped her antibiotic. The next day the patient stopped scratching.[2]

Masturbation (sexual self-stimulation) is a normal means of sexual expression when no partner is available. However, some patients masturbate excessively, which may indicate serious underlying problems. Occasionally, some people masturbate publicly. In the nursing home, masturbation should be discouraged in public places. The feelings and sensitivities of all residents and staff must be considered.

Masturbation may also be a form of sensory stimulation when nothing else is available. One patient in a nursing home masturbated openly and frequently throughout the day. One day a nursing assistant who was playing a ball game with some nearby residents, accidently threw the ball toward this man. He caught it and threw it back. He joined the group and began playing ball and cards. He very rarely, if ever, was seen masturbating again in public.

Many people are satisfied with alternatives to physical sexual expression, such as talking, laughing, playing games, and dancing with people of the opposite sex. They should be given opportunities to do these things. They should have the chance to feel the warmth of another body, perhaps a child's or a pet's. They should be encouraged to form new friendships and find new companions. Socials and group discussions about books, plants, or travel, for example) can be very helpful in this regard.

Nursing homes are not known for the privacy that they provide for their residents. Nursing assistants must respect their patients' privacy as much as possible, however. They should knock and wait for an answer when a patient's door is closed. Marriage among the elderly is becoming more common and even occurs in nursing homes occasionally. Long-married couples frequently enter nursing homes together. In view of this, more thought should be given to accommodating married couples in the long-term care setting.

SAFETY AND SECURITY

Most people in nursing homes have failing health. They need to be prevented from contracting any further illness. They need to have their own water cup, tissues, wash basin, soap, towel, and washcloth. Items should not be interchanged between patients. Nursing assistants must wash their hands with soap and water when going from one patient to the next. Special soap and paper towels should be available for this purpose.

As people get older, they have more accidental injuries and can be greatly incapacitated by them. Many accidents are due to the physical changes of aging.

Impairment of Vision

In old age, people tend to become farsighted. Because of changes in the lens of the eye, the farsighted person must hold books farther away in order to read them. Sight also becomes dimmer in old age. Most aging people need brighter lights for reading and sewing. Those with cataracts, however, cannot stand the glare of a bright light. As we grow older, we see less well in the dark. It takes longer for older people to see when they go from a lighted room to a dark room. For this reason, a night light is essential in every room and bathroom in the nursing home.

In order to help a person with a visual loss, try to discover what that loss is. How much can he see—your face, its shape, its features, or only a shadow? Is his side (peripheral) vision impaired? Some patients have tunnel vision. This means they can only see a very small area directly in front of them. It is as though they were wearing a mask with very small openings to see through. These people are often accused of pretending that they can't see. For example, Mrs. Rico can pick up a piece of dust from her pillow and can spot a pin that has dropped on the floor, but she can't find the bathroom or her bed. Some people who have had strokes may be blind in half of each eye. For example, the inner aspect of the right eye and the outer aspect of the left eye may be blind. Such patients miss half of what they are looking at. They often eat the food from one side of their tray only. Mr. Faust is blind in the right side of both eyes. He always left food on the right side of his tray until he was reminded to turn his head to the right.

When caring for a person with a visual loss, tell him who you are as you enter the room, and let him know when you are leaving. When talking with him, position your face in his best line of sight. Get close enough so that he can, if possible, identify your features. Keep the person's room in order, *his* order. Do not move things where he will not be able to find them. Make certain floors are not cluttered with items that can be tripped over, and wipe up wet spots that could be slipped on.

If the older person with impaired vision has prescribed eyeglasses, he should wear them. If he objects to wearing them, find out what the problem is and have it corrected. Fluorescent tapes around light switches and door handles, large silhouettes of men or women on bathroom doors, large print on signs, books with large type, and talking records are among the many devices that can help people who have trouble seeing.

Hearing Loss

With age, hearing is progressively lost, often for the high-pitched sounds. At first, this loss is not noticed because normal conversation does not contain very many high-pitched sounds. In time, the higher notes of normal speech—the Ch, , Th, T and P sounds—can no longer be heard. This interferes with understanding what is said. If one cannot hear these sounds, speech sounds garbled and the patient has to guess what is being said. People with this hearing loss may confuse one word for another and respond to what they *thought* they heard. They may begin to think people are talking about them. Often they give you the impression that they do not hear you, but when you increase the loudness of your voice they say, "You don't have to shout. I'm not deaf." Although they only hear some of the sounds, those sounds are often as loud to them as to the person with normal hearing. Another type of hearing loss in the aged is when *all* sounds seem less loud than before. In addition to this loss, some people may not be able to hear the high-pitched sounds.

When you wish to talk with a resident with a hearing loss, touch him to get his attention. Position yourself face to face with the person at his eye-level. If he is lying in bed, bring your face close to the level of the mattress. If he is in a wheelchair, get in front of the chair and squat down. Know how severe the loss is and if it involves one or both ears. Speak slowly and clearly. Do not shout. Have paper and pencil available and use it to write down what you want to communicate, if necessary. Make an attempt to communicate regularly throughout the day. Too often people who are hard of hearing are avoided. Often they do not get the information and explanations they need. Often they are not encouraged to attend social functions.

Many older people who have lost their hearing late in life will attempt to lip-read or will be willing to learn to lip-read. However, nursing assistants should encourage older people who have prescribed hearing aids to use them. It does take time to adjust to them and patients often become discouraged and leave them in their tables. Nursing assistants should know how to operate, maintain, and clean them. If instructions are not available, a local hearing aid dealer can supply them. All patients' ears should be cleaned often. Ear wax can seriously interfere with hearing.

Skin Deterioration

The skin of many elderly persons becomes thin and dry and loses elasticity. There is less protective tissue under the skin. The skin should be washed with mild soap and sometimes with no soap. It should be lubricated with lotion. If there is a break in the skin, report it to a nurse and give special care and attention to the area. Keeping your patients' hair, face, hands, and feet well-groomed is as important to their self-image as the clothing they wear.

Perception of Pain

With increasing age, perception of pain, heat, and cold decreases. You must be careful to avoid giving applications that are too hot or too cold. Do not expect that all of your older patients will complain of pain when something is seriously wrong with them. Nursing home residents have been known to have heart attacks without chest pain and appendicitis without abdominal pain. Use all of your senses and be constantly alert for signs that may indicate a problem.

Sense of Balance and Reaction Time

The older person's balance may be affected. This may occur when the head is turned too quickly or when the patient stands quickly after lying or sitting. It is important that older persons change positions slowly.

With advancing age, reaction time usually slows down. The older person may realize what he must do, but may take longer to do it. He may have to think out more consciously the steps of each task. If he is hurried, he may fumble or have an accident. Allow plenty of time for your patients to do things. Give directions one at a time. Demonstrate as well as tell how to do things.

Nurturing a Sense of Security

Older people feel more secure when they can help themselves. Nursing assistants who believe they are showing their concern for their patients by doing everything for them may, instead, be causing irreparable damage. More caring is shown by having the patience to give your patients time in which to do anything they are capable of doing themselves. Not only does this help them remain flexible and strong, but it also makes them feel better about themselves. Those who have been independent all their lives may feel shame at needing help from someone else. When they must ask for help, give it in a willing and pleasant manner.

Elderly residents of nursing homes need places they can call their own. Each needs his own territory, even if it is only two or three feet surrounding a bed. Each needs his own belongings around him. The belongings help him keep a sense of identity and stay oriented. Older people need to be allowed clutter on the bedside stand and in the bed (within the limits of safety, of course—food that would attract bugs or objects that might be harmful should be discouraged). They should be allowed to place these objects in any order they prefer. Then they can reach for them and find them easily. Older people need some sort of stimulation for their eyes and ears, and these familiar objects help provide this.

Devices to enhance patient safety should include beds with wheels that lock and that can be placed in both high and low positions, siderails on beds, grab rails in bathrooms and halls, nonskid mats in bathtubs and showers, and wheelchairs with regularly maintained brakes and tires.

LOVE AND BELONGING, SELF-ESTEEM, SELF-REALIZATION

Everyone, including the elderly, needs interaction with other people of all ages. Our society tends to segregate the elderly. Many of them see only those who are about their own age. The stories and complaints they hear are all too familiar. Each nursing home should have some means by which its residents can have opportunities to talk with people of all ages. Families and friends should be encouraged to visit and to take patients home for visits.

Older people need friends or people whom they can rely on and trust, people who care about them. *Significant others* are those people in a person's life who confirm the fact that that he is a useful, respected person. Nursing assistants should know who the significant others are in their patients' lives and encourage them to talk about them. Someone in the nursing home may want to take the position of significant other in one patient's life. This is particularly important for the person who will not leave the long-term care facility. The responsibilities of this position may be no more than a daily greeting, a show of concern, and a word of encouragement to the patient. But this may be extremely meaningful to that person. Sometimes the nursing assistant can introduce two people with similar interests. This small gesture may begin a significant relationship.

Satisfying Use of Time

Many of the generation which is now elderly grew up with the belief that having leisure time is sinful. Forced retirement may have introduced or reinforced feelings of worthlessness and uselessness. Leisure-time programs or activities planned for the elderly may be their only means of socializing, or of doing something that helps them be themselves and keep their personalities intact. But programs that don't consider the interests of the elderly people participating in them will be useless.

Having Direction and Purpose

The person who enters a nursing home often feels frightened and devastated. He may seem to lose all sense of a future. The nursing assistant, who is closest to the patient, has the opportunity to find out what the patient really wants to do. If he could do one thing, what would it be? Possibly this is the direction toward which nearly all of the care of the person should go. Many elderly patients who have had strokes have relearned to dress themselves, and to walk, motivated by a goal such as being able once again to go outdoors, see the grass, feed the birds, or garden. If the patient and those taking care of him have the same goal in mind, it can be more easily achieved.

Venting Feelings Without Shame

In some nursing homes, the staff resent any complaints or criticism by patients. But residents should be permitted to express their feelings and to talk about themselves and their situation. For the good of all, however, some limits have to be set as to what is an acceptable show of feelings.

Making Decisions

Wherever and whenever possible, residents in nursing homes should be allowed to make decisions about themselves and their care. Regimenting residents in long-term care facilities often contributes to increased dependence, loss of self-esteem, and decline. We all need to feel that we have some control over our lives. When we do not have this feeling, we become apathetic—"If nobody else cares, why should I?"

Some patients are not able to make decisions for themselves. Nursing assistants must observe very carefully how patients exercise judgment when they are given the opportunity to make decisions. The man who insists on taking his wheelchair down steps obviously should not be allowed to travel alone in his chair, or should travel alone only where there are no steps.

Some older people have good judgment except when it comes to setting limits on themselves. They may be so proud or independent that they overtire themselves despite warning symptoms like shortness of breath or pain. These people need help to understand some of the changes that come with increasing age and to learn to recognize their limits.

Nearly all patients, however, even those with poor judgment in one area or another, need the freedom to make some choices about what they will do. When you give a patient a choice, you help him gain a feeling of control. But whenever you give a choice, such as whether to watch TV or to go to the recreation room, you must follow through and allow your patient the choice he makes. If you do not, your patient will lose trust in you.

Having New Experiences and New Learning Opportunities

Older people should have the opportunity to learn new skills and gain new information. They need the stimulation that we all need to make life interesting (speakers, films, groups). Many feel that there is nothing new in the world for them because they are no longer useful. Many feel that because of their age they can no longer learn. Thus, they themselves are victims of the stereotypes about the aged. When faced with a new learning experience, older people often are afraid of failure. A younger person would approach learning how to knit by thinking about having a finished scarf. The older person might approach learning to knit nervously, afraid of being humiliated. All new learning experiences should be begun slowly, one step at a time, at the patient's pace. Learning experiences should be planned so that the simplest task comes first, and so that the learner will be successful.

When you teach a stroke patient to dress himself, begin with one piece of clothing. If it is a shirt, start by having the patient put it on his lap correctly. Then show him how to put the affected arm in the sleeve and how to pull the sleeve up over the arm—one step at a time.

When you help a person begin to feed himself again, start by placing him in a normal sitting position. His feet should be flat on the floor. He should be close enough to the table to be able to see and reach the food. Find out his food likes and dislikes beforehand. Offer him something he likes. If the silverware is difficult for him to handle, have him begin to feed himself with finger foods such as a hamburger, a cracker, or a cookie. You may have to give him very specific instructions about how to pick up the food and lift it to his mouth. If his silverware needs to be adjusted in some way (perhaps with a longer handle or an attached strap) so that he can use it more easily, ask the nurse or occupational therapy consultant how this can be done.

Passing Wisdom or Experience on to the Younger Generation

Listening to the advice and experiences of old people should be part of everyone's life. Nursing assistants will find their jobs much more rewarding if they listen, question, and try to learn from their older patients. These patients should be given the opportunity to interact with children, teenagers, and young adults. They should be encouraged to pass on the valuable information they have gained throughout their lives. In some communities, Boy Scouts and Girl Scouts "adopt a grandparent" in a nursing home and visit the "grandparent" regularly.

Spiritual Needs

The spiritual part of man is the center of his being. As many people grow older, they take a second look at what religion means to them. Often they find it gives them strength and courage when their bodies and those around them fail them. It gives them hope for the present and helps them prepare for a meaningful death.

Those who take care of the elderly must learn to accept and tolerate all religious beliefs. They must not try to force their own beliefs on others. Find out what your patients' beliefs are and in what way they practice them. When your patients want someone to give them spiritual support or guidance, or wish to attend religious services, make sure their requests are made known to the proper person on the staff.

SUMMARY

All human beings have the same basic needs. These cannot really be separated from one another and put into convenient pigeonholes. You can't separate the person and his thoughts from his body. If he is uncomfortable in one or the other or both, this is a signal that he needs help.

You cannot say, "Now I'm going to respond to Mr. Neal's need for self-esteem," or, "Now I'm going to respond to his need for activity." The action of giving a bath may be the means by which you can talk, listen, and build trust with your patient. Helping him get out of bed and walk to a chair not only maintains his mobility, but builds his self-esteem.

REFERENCES

[1] Abraham Maslow, *Motivation and Personality* (New York: Harper and Brothers, Publishers, 1971). **NOTE:** This is the author's understanding or interpretation of Maslow's writing.

[2] Dorothea Jaeger and Leo W. Simmons, *The Aged Ill* (New York: Appleton-Century-Crofts, 1970), p. 85.

DISCUSSION QUESTIONS

1. How might a regular occasion for dressing up be arranged for residents in your home?
2. How could your facility be changed to make it more like a home?
3. How can you help an older person who is restricted to his bed or chair keep active?
4. How can the environment of your nursing home be changed to prevent injuries and accidents?
5. How can too much help or TLC hurt your older patient?
6. How do you respect your older patients' right to privacy?
7. What opportunities do patients in your institution have to be with people of other age groups?
8. What opportunities do patients in your nursing home have to pass on their wisdom and experience to younger adults and children?

9. How can your patients have opportunities to learn something new?

10. To which religious groups do your patients belong? Discuss some of the major beliefs and customs of these groups.

11. List the basic needs of man. Think of a patient whose needs you must fulfill. How can this patient be helped to meet these needs himself?

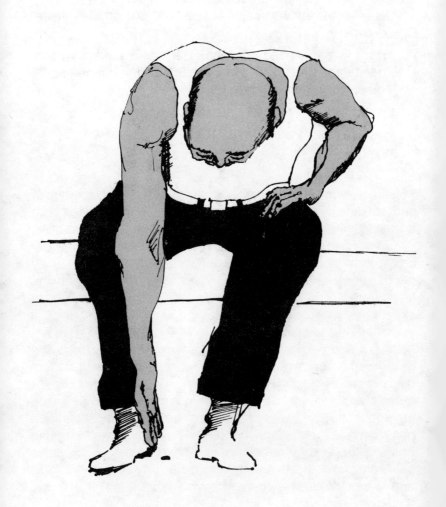

4

Being a Helping and Caring Person

You are a member of the helping professions, a special group of people who care for people in need. This means you need both a knowledge of human nature and a great deal of compassion.

Older people are often brought to the nursing home because they have needs they cannot meet themselves. They need to be helped and cared for. This does not make them any less human or valuable as human beings. It is their right to expect help and care.

Nursing assistants are people who help people. Being a helping person does not only mean doing physical things like giving baths and making beds. It means helping your patient help himself as much as possible, helping him meet his needs. It means talking to him and allowing him to tell you what his needs are so that he can better cope with another day. It could mean being a friend to him. Older people, particularly those in nursing homes, desperately need a helping, caring person. Besides being old and ill, their situations in life often involve many losses and fears. This leaves them little energy for coping.

54

Establishing a helping relationship in which you and the patient respect one another and work toward a common goal takes effort. This effort is worthwhile because the helping relationship is satisfying to both you and the patient. The patient gains more self-esteem and independence, and both you and the patient gain more self-understanding.

BUILDING TRUST

To establish a helping relationship, you must act in such a manner that your patient can trust you. It takes a long time to really trust someone, to build a trusting relationship.

Be Honest

To build a trusting relationship with your patient, you must *be honest* not only in what you say to him but in your feelings toward him. Sometimes telling him that his actions make you angry will help him. Just because you are angry at his actions does not mean you dislike him.

You cannot be honest with your patients if you think you must humor them all the time. For example, you shouldn't say, "Everything is OK," or "It's going to be all right," if such is not the case.

Also, you can't expect to be smiling and happy all the time you are with your patients. Elderly people are living in nursing homes as they would in their own homes. They expect people who care for them to express different emotions at appropriate times.

Have Patience

You must *be patient* if you are to build trust. In the long-term care setting, many actions performed by nursing assistants are repeated over and over without any apparent results. Turning and repositioning a patient every two hours day and night may only mean more work to someone who does not understand that doing this prevents bedsores and stiffening of the joints. Ask a nurse what your actions are supposed to accomplish and what signs would indicate whether these goals are being achieved. For example, while you are turning a person, you may see a reddened area on his hip that does not go away after he has not lain on it for half an hour. You should report this to a nurse so that a new schedule of turning can be arranged.

It is true that older patients do not recover from injuries and emotional upsets as quickly as younger ones do. But if they are cared for properly, they *do* recover. A break in the skin of an older person may take weeks to heal, but carelessness in treating it may prevent it from ever healing.

Older people need more time in which to do things. Many have long-established ways of performing the tasks of daily living. Allow them to do it their way.

Some older people may repeat what they do or say many times. Try to understand why this is so. Listen and observe.

Be Consistent

To build trust, you must *be consistent.* Do what you said you would do. If you promised to come back to a resident's room by a particular time for a particular purpose, do it. If you cannot keep your promise, at least go to the resident and tell him when you will be back, or have someone else give him a message from you.

Explain What You Are Going To Do

To build trust, you must *explain what you are going to do* before you do it. Whenever you move an older person or any part of his body, tell him what you are about to do. People quickly begin to feel less human when they are rolled, pushed, pulled, and lifted without any explanation or words of warning. When you see a patient who is new to you, tell him who you are and how long you will be with him. Also, tell him if he has any appointments scheduled or specimens due within the next few hours. Telling him this ahead of time will make it easier for you to get the specimen or less likely that he will be late for his appointment. Older people need time to adjust to a change and time to prepare for an appointment. They are more easily flustered when they are hurried than when they are given plenty of time.

Allow Patients to Express Their Feelings

In order to build trust, you must let your patients *express their feelings* without taking their remarks personally and without trying "to get even." People living in nursing homes sometimes need to be angry and shout. Usually, no one person or incident is entirely responsible for the patient's anger, but usually only one person is picked to hear about it. Sometimes people working in nursing homes unconsciously punish patients for behavior that they do not like or understand. They do this in many little ways, such as giving the patient little or no attention, not helping him eat or get out of bed, or making him wait for water to drink or a bedpan or assistance to the bathroom. Withholding these things from patients can be devastating to them and will destroy any future relationships with them.

Be Nonjudgmental

In order to build trust you must *not judge the other person.* You must not place a value (good or bad, right or wrong) on his actions or words. You must accept different religious practices, life styles, eating habits, dressing habits, and so forth, and try to understand them. Some people laugh at anything they are not used to, such as a different way of speaking or dressing or a different hair length. Or they call it bad or wrong. You cannot do this if you want to help your patients. You must be warm, accepting, and understanding.

Show That You Care For Your Patients

In order to build trust you must *show that you care for your patients.* All human beings need a sense of belonging, a sense that someone cares, that they are recognized for themselves and have worth. Elderly people have these same needs. They need someone who cares. When someone shows that he cares, it gives value to the other's existence. When you show an older person that you care, it gives him a reason to live. Caring may make the difference between striving to live and giving up and dying.

Caring is an attitude of the heart. It is a positive feeling toward someone or something. The many dictionary definitions include "having interest in," "being fond of," "having concern for," "being protecting," "guarding or watching over."

Caring for another person is helping him or her grow. This definition, which is particularly meaningful to those working with the elderly, is from a book called *On Caring* by Milton Mayeroff. Here "growing" does not mean physical growth, but learning to become more comfortable with oneself and one's surroundings. It also means learning how to adapt one's life and how it is lived to one's changing body and circumstances. In this sense, caring, to those working in nursing homes, is helping elderly people meet their needs. It is helping them find new ways to help themselves.

> . . . I experience what I care for as having worth in its own right. In caring I experience the other as having strengths and the need to grow. . . I do not experience being needed by the other as a relationship that gives me power over [him] and provides me with something to dominate, but rather as a kind of trust. It is as if I had been entrusted with the care of the other in a way that is the opposite of possessing and manipulating [him] as I please. . . In helping the other grow I do not impose my own direction; rather I allow the direction of the other's growth to guide what I do, to help determine how I am to respond and what is relevant to such a response. . . Any direction that I may give the other is governed by my respect for his integrity and is intended to further his growth. . .[1]

You can show caring in many ways. According to Mayeroff, there are certain "ingredients" of caring. First, you must *know your patients* and let them get to know you.

I must know who the other is, what his powers and limitations are, what his needs are. . . I must know how to respond to his needs and what my own powers and limitations are.[2]

This means not only knowing your patients' names and faces, but knowing them as individuals. It means getting them to talk about themselves so that you know their likes and dislikes, their religious beliefs, and their former occupations. It means knowing how they normally look and act, and their daily schedules. It means checking the nursing care plans and nursing notes daily for information that may help you understand why your patients feel and act as they do. It means knowing that Mrs. Ortiz needs to stay in bed for at least an hour after waking in the morning because of her stiff arthritic joints. It means knowing that her roommate has a very strict morning routine for washing and dressing which she starts at 7:00 a.m., and that she becomes angry when this is interfered with. Knowing your patients means planning your assignments around their needs and not your convenience.

Second, you must *evaluate* your action each time for each patient to determine whether it has helped or not, and you must change the action if it has not helped.

To determine whether I am caring, I must not only observe what I do, feel and intend, but I must also observe whether the other is growing as a result of what I do.[3]

Mrs. Nielsen has severe arthritis that interferes with movement of her shoulders, elbows, wrists, and fingers. It is hard for her to get food to her mouth without dropping her fork. Consequently, she eats very little and is losing weight. Mary LaSalle, a nursing assistant, attempted to help Mrs. Nielsen by feeding her. But Mrs. Nielsen felt humiliated by this, refused to eat, and began to cry. Miss LaSalle realized that she must find some better way of helping Mrs. Nielsen feed herself. She asked the nurse about the possibility of obtaining specially designed silverware that could be secured to Mrs. Nielsen's hand with a strap.

Mary LaSalle evaluated her action (feeding her patient) by watching how it was responded to (Mrs. Nielsen refused to eat and cried). When Miss LaSalle realized she wasn't helping Mrs. Nielsen, she decided to try another approach.

Third, you must *help your patients grow* by looking for their strengths. Then you can plan how their strengths can be used to make up for their weaknesses. Try to find out what each person can do for himself despite his handicaps.

I must see the other as [he] is and not as I would like [him] to be or feel [he] must be. If I am to help the other to grow, I must respond to [his] changing needs. If I can only see what I would like to see, I will not be able to see the other as [he] really is.[4]

Caring is making reasonable demands of your elderly patients, encouraging them to do for themselves no matter how long it takes. Setting and combing a patient's hair may be fun, but if the patient can do it herself, she should do it. Do not deny her your companionship or some assistance, but think how much she will benefit by moving her arms to her head, looking at herself in the mirror, and seeing the results of her efforts. However, when a patient really needs help, you should give it willingly. When a person cannot get to a commode or toilet and must use a bedpan, caring means giving and taking the pan as quickly as possible and not making a fuss over it. It is assuring the person that this activity is one of the many you perform throughout the day. It is making him feel that you are concerned about his comfort and safety and would be more concerned if he did not call for the pan.

A caring person must have *humility*. You must be yourself, know your own strengths and weaknesses, and realize that you can learn from others, including your elderly patients.

Never forget the existence of the person for whom you are caring. When two nursing assistants are working together, they should not carry on a private conversation that leaves out the patient. They should not wash a person as though he were an object while carrying on a personal conversation.

No matter how childish your patients' behavior may seem at times, do not forget that they are adults who have experienced adult lives. Everyone wants some protection and babying, but overprotection and overbabying make people feel useless and inadequate.

A caring person must also *care for himself.* Caring for yourself is reflected in your appearance—neat hair and clothing, clean face and hands and nails. Caring for yourself is also conveyed by how you act toward others. If you care for yourself you will respect others and not be condescending, manipulative, punishing, angry, or indifferent.

Caring can be defined in many ways. It is a feeling that is expressed in the way you perform your everyday tasks. It is reflected in how you look, how you speak, and how well you perform your duties. It also shows in how you touch. *Touching* can communicate caring better than anything else to confused, blind, or psychotic patients.

We all know the difference between a rough and a gentle touch. A rough touch usually indicates anger or being in a hurry or just not caring. In contrast, a gentle touch is used for someone special, someone whom you wish to please.

Caring is *allowing privacy.* This means preventing exposure of a person who is washing, dressing, or toileting by providing a bath blanket or curtains around the bed, or by closing the door. It means respecting a person's private belongings, handling them carefully and respectfully, and not discarding anything without getting permission.

Caring means *accepting* people despite changes in their behavior and attitude toward you. It means letting them know that you will not "give up" on them and that you are trying to help them overcome their problem.

Caring is a special quality expressed by people regardless of their skills or training. Having this quality gives meaning to all the things nursing assistants do. It brings satisfaction to you as well as to your patients.

Two important aspects of caring and helping are *communication* and *observation.* These will be discussed in following chapters.

SUMMARY

You are an important member of the helping professions. But becoming a helping person takes effort. It involves building trusting relationships with your patients. In order to build trust you must be honest, have patience, be consistent, explain what you are doing, allow patients to express their feelings, be non-judgmental, and show that you care.

Caring is the essential "ingredient" for becoming a really good geriatric nursing assistant. It requires understanding of and consideration for the needs of elderly persons living in the nursing home setting.

REFERENCES

[1]Milton Mayeroff, *On Caring* (New York: Harper and Row, Publishers, Inc., 1971), pp. 6-8.
[2]Ibid., p. 13.
[3]Ibid., p. 39.
[4]Ibid., p. 19.

DISCUSSION QUESTIONS

1. What are the "ingredients" of caring? How has the use of any of these helped one of your patients?

2. How can reading the nursing care plan help you know your patients better?

3. When should you touch? Is your touch gentle or rough?

4. Have you had patients on whom you wanted to "give up"? If you did give up, why did you?

5. How can you show that you care about yourself?

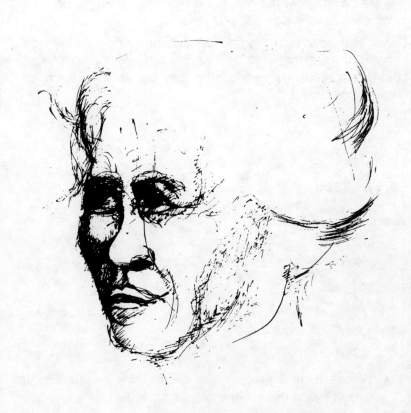

HOW CAN I CREATE A HELPING RELATIONSHIP?

1. Can I be in some way which will be seen by the other person as trustworthy, as dependable or consistent?

2. Can I be expressive enough as a person that what I am will be communicated without understanding?

3. Can I let myself experience positive attitudes toward this other person—attitudes of warmth, caring, liking, interest, respect?

4. Can I be strong enough as a person to be separate from the other? Can I be a sturdy respecter of my own feelings, my own needs, as well as his? Can I own, and if need be, express my own feelings as something belonging to me and separate from his feelings? Am I strong enough in my own separateness that I will not be downcast by his depression, frightened by his fear, not engulfed by his dependency? Is my inner self hardy enough to realize that I am not destroyed by his anger, taken over by his need for dependence, nor enslaved by his love, but that I exist separate from him with feelings and rights of my own?

5. Am I secure enough within myself to permit him his separateness? Can I permit him to be what he is—honest or deceitful, infantile or adult, despairing or over-confident? Can I give him the freedom to be? Or do I feel that he should follow my advice, or remain somewhat dependent on me, or mold himself after me?

6. Can I let myself enter into the world of his feelings and personal meanings and see them as he does? Without judging it? Can I be sensitive so that I do not trample on meanings which are precious to him? Can I sense his world accurately enough to catch not only the meanings of his experience which are obvious to him, but those meanings which are only implicit, which he sees only dimly or as confusion? Can I help him with these too?

7. Can I be acceptant of each side of this other person which he presents to me? Can I receive him as he is? Can I communicate this attitude? Or can I only receive him conditionally, acceptant of some parts of his feelings and silently or openly disapproving of other aspects?

8. Can I be sensitive enough to his world that I will not threaten him?

9. Can I help him to be free from fear of the judgments of others?

10. Can I meet this other individual as a person who is in the process of becoming, or will I be bound by his past and by my past?

From Carl R. Rogers, *On Becoming A Person* (Boston: Houghton Mifflin Company, 1961), pp. 50-55.

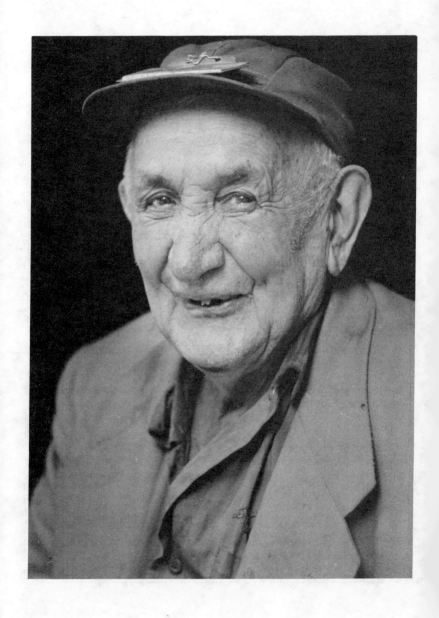

5

Communication

Communicating with your patients and allowing them to communicate with you is the key to being a successful helping person. Communication is all the ways by which we try to influence other people.[1] It is the interaction between people. It is sharing ourselves with others—our feelings, ideas, beliefs. It is attempting to "put ourselves in other peoples' shoes" and "see through their eyes."

THE FIVE ELEMENTS OF COMMUNICATION

In order for communication to occur, five elements must be present. If one of these elements is missing, communication cannot occur. These five elements are:[2]

A *sender.* This is a source of information, which may be a living person or an inanimate object such as a tape recorder, television, radio, or record player.

A *message.* This is the information which is to be sent.

A *channel of transmission.* If the message is spoken, it travels via sound waves to the listener. If the message is written or gestured, it requires light.

A receiver. Someone or something "hears" the message.

A response. If the receiver is a person, he or she tries to understand and respond to the message. If the receiver is a machine, its response may be the click of a button which turns on a tape recorder or makes some sort of electronic recording of the message.

When a nursing assistant (sender) says to a resident, "Your doctor will be coming this afternoon" (message via sound waves), and the resident (receiver) answers, "Good. I've got a lot to say to him" (response), communication has occurred. However, if the resident answers, "I didn't expect my daughter until tomorrow," one element of communication, an appropriate response, is lacking. So communication has not occurred.

VERBAL AND NONVERBAL COMMUNICATION

There are two kinds of communication—verbal and nonverbal. Verbal communication depends on language to transmit the message, and it is usually a voluntary act, such as speaking and writing. Nonverbal communication does not depend on words. It expresses feelings or emotions in other ways, such as:

- Facial expressions (a smile; a frown; a twist of the mouth; raised eyebrows).

- Gestures and body movements (a shrug of the shoulder; hand movements).

- Posture of the body (hunching over; standing straight).

- Tone of voice (sarcastic; friendly).

- Smells (the odor of excrement; the fragrance of cologne).
- Space (the distance between two people as they talk; how close a nursing assistant gets to her patient).
- Silence (approving; sympathetic; hostile).
- Touch (gentle; rough).

People send nonverbal messages all the time. Often they are unaware that they are doing so.

When verbal and nonverbal messages are contradictory, people tend to believe the nonverbal message. When a resident says he is fine with a frown on his face, you probably suspect something is wrong.

HOW HEARING AND LISTENING DIFFER

Nursing assistants and their patients need to be continuously communicating throughout the day. But just because they are talking does not mean they are communicating. Two common communication problems are: 1) that the nursing assistant does not receive the patient's message, and 2) that the patient does not receive the nursing assistant's message.

One of the ways that you can miss your patient's message is by not listening. *Hearing* is a passive awareness of sound. It is an involuntary action. To hear, you need only use your ears. *Listening* is an active, conscientious attempt to hear what the message is and what it means. It is a voluntary act and requires concentration and close attention to what is being said and done.[3] To listen well and to be sure to get the complete message you must look directly at the person who is speaking and you must be alert. It is difficult to really listen when you are tired. Try to put yourself in the patient's place, but remember that you and he or she do not necessarily think alike. Most of all, try to put aside your own prejudices and values. They will only get in your way and cause you to misinterpret the message.

BARRIERS THAT PREVENT COMMUNICATION

Another way that you can miss your patient's message is by putting up "barriers" that can prevent him from expressing himself. Some of these barriers include:

- *Changing the subject.* When you respond to a person's statement by changing the subject, you take the lead in the conversation and block the individual's attempts to discuss what he wishes.

- *Giving your own opinion about the person and his situation without being asked.* Your opinion may "turn him off." He may just want to talk about his opinion.

- *Belittling a person's feelings.* This suggests that he and his problem are not important. It implies that you are not interested in him as an individual.

- *Seeming to be too busy.* You may be implying that you have too little time to bother with the person.

- *Jumping to conclusions before you know the entire story.*

- *Giving false or inappropriate reassurances.* When you respond to a patient by saying, "Everything is going to be

all right," or "You're not going to die," without any knowledge of the person's condition, or with the knowledge that
what you said is not true, you stop that person from talking
further and from expressing his feelings.

- *Causing fear of an unpleasant response.* If the person who
calls for assistance is greeted with a sarcastic "Now what
do you want," he will be less likely to make his needs
known.

OTHER REASONS WHY MESSAGES ARE MISSED

Not only do you sometimes miss your patients' messages,
but they may also miss yours. Many elderly and not so elderly
people miss messages because they are preoccupied with their
thoughts and feelings. Another major reason they may completely miss or misinterpret what is said to them is that their
hearing or seeing may be impaired. Also, their thinking pro-
cesses may have slowed so that they need a more slowly
spoken message and more time in which to respond to it.

Aphasia

Another reason why your patient may not respond to your
message is that he may have a language disorder, an aphasia,
due to a stroke. This disorder may interfere with his ability to
understand and/or use language in speaking, writing, or reading. Not only does each person with aphasia have individual

problem areas, but the severity of the problem differs from person to person. Some people may be able to understand only written language or gestures. Some may be able to comprehend only spoken language. Some may not be able to understand at all. Others may be able to comprehend, but not be able to express themselves by writing or by gesturing. Many try to communicate but have trouble finding the right words. They may know what they want to say, but their sentences sound scrambled. Some may repeat the same word or phrase over and over again in an attempt to communicate. These may be words such as "yes," "no," "I can't," "I don't know." Swearing may be another form of automatic speech. This is embarrassing to the staff and the patient's family, but it is a means of expression for a person with no other emotional outlet.

If your patient has any one of these variations of aphasia, there will be a problem with communication. Try to find out what the problem is. Try to establish communication by the best possible means (gestures, flash cards, pencil and paper). Give the person plenty of time to respond to what you say or do. Encourage his efforts at speech or communication, but do not pressure him.

COMMUNICATING EFFECTIVELY

You can communicate more effectively with your elderly patients by:

Showing an interest in talking with them, but not prying.

Allowing time for talking. The best time for this may be

while you are doing something for and with the patient. It is a time when, no matter what you are doing, your goal should be to have the patient talk if he wants to.

Pacing yourself to the speed at which your patient talks. If your patient speaks slowly, speak a little slower than he does. This will allow him time to think about what you've said and to answer you. Reword sentences that seem difficult, using the person's own words or jargon. Ask only one question at a time and get an answer before asking another.

Trying to get at the person's eye level and staying within his sight. This makes it easier for him or her to see your expression and your lips. Patients with hearing losses may try to read lips if they can see them. If you stand too far away or too much to the side they may not be able to see you. At night, hold the flashlight so that your face is visible to the patient.

Exploring the reasons why communication is not occurring, if this is so. There have been patients who have come into nursing homes appearing withdrawn and confused. These people did not speak and were thought to be aphasic. Later it was found that they could speak and understand if others would speak their language. They spoke foreign languages.

Remembering that when you communicate you are not only conveying words, but also your attitudes and feelings about yourself and others.

Reminiscence–a Form of Communication

Reminiscence is a very important part of the aging process. At one time it was thought that people who frequently reviewed their lives were getting "senile" and/or losing touch with reality. This is no longer believed to be true. It is now thought that the life review is a way of preparing oneself for death. By going over his past the older person tries to resolve problems and come to the conclusion that his life was a satisfying one. Some people cannot come to this conclusion and become depressed. Others are not entirely satisfied, but are able to accept their lives.

Some people review their lives by telling a story about someone else. Some may seem to be complaining, "I should have. . ." Some may seem to be talking to themselves. Many just "remember when. . ." The best thing that you can do for these people is to listen. If you do not have time to listen to the whole story, tell the older person why you have to leave and when you will be back.

Listening thoughtfully as an older person tells his story again and again may be difficult. Yet, for the older person, another person listening to him or her is better than medicine.

SUMMARY

In order to be a helping person, you must learn to communicate with your patients. You must encourage them to talk and you must listen very carefully to what they are saying.

REFERENCES

[1]Garland K. Lewis, *Nurse-Patient Communication* (Dubuque, Iowa: Wm. C. Brown Company Publishers, 1969), p. 8.

[2]James K. Skipper, Jr., and Robert C. Leonard, *Social Interaction and Patient Care* (Philadelphia: J.B. Lippincott Company, 1965), p. 52.

[3]Garland, *op. cit.,* p. 33.

[4]Robert N. Butler, and Myrna I. Lewis, *Aging and Mental Health, Positive Psychosocial Approaches* (St. Louis: The C.V. Mosby Company, 1973), pp. 43-44.

DISCUSSION QUESTIONS

1. How well do you listen? After a five-minute conversation with one of your patients, can you write down most of what the patient said?

2. What are some nonverbal signs that you received from your patients today? What do you think they meant?

3. How can you communicate with a person who cannot speak?

4. What are some signs that would indicate that a person has a hearing or seeing problem? Do any of your patients have any of these signs?

5. How can your personal problems interfere with your ability to communicate?

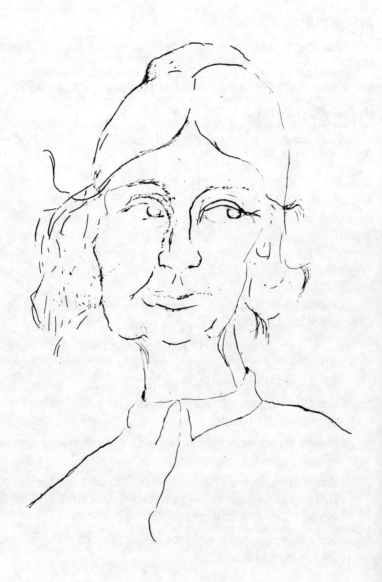

6

Observation

Of all the helping people in nursing homes, nursing assistants are the ones who are closest to patients for the longest periods of time. This gives them a tremendous opportunity to observe. The more they know about their patients, the more meaningful are their observations.

Observation is an important nursing tool that needs to be sharpened by practice every day. It requires a highly conscious awareness of one's surroundings. It requires the use of all of one's senses—seeing, hearing, smelling, and touching.

SEEING

Seeing is probably the first sense one thinks of in connection with observing. However, you can *see* something and not really *observe* it. You can be aware that the floor is wet, but until you determine what color the fluid is and if it has an odor, you have no way of understanding what it is. If you are *only seeing* (allowing light to enter your eye and form an image), you are not *observing*. You must look and think about what you are seeing and what it means. When you do this, you are observing.

Kathy O'Neill, a nursing assistant, was helping Mr. Mancini, a new patient, undress and get ready for bed. She noticed many bruises on his legs. When she asked him how he got the bruises, he said he didn't know. Miss O'Neill immediately reported the bruises to her charge nurse. The nurse knew that Mr. Mancini was taking an anticoagulant medicine to prevent the blood from clotting as quickly as normal. She also knew that too much of the medication can cause bleeding into the tissues. The bruises were small areas of bleeding into the tissues. By reporting this sign immediately, Miss O'Neill prevented Mr. Mancini from bleeding more seriously. When his medication was reduced, the bruises disappeared.

HEARING

Hearing is a sense that can be made more useful with practice. On page 69 in this text, the difference between hearing and listening was explained. You must listen in order to observe accurately. Hearing involves being aware of a sound. Listening involves hearing the sound and trying to understand what it means.

While helping Mr. Snyder with his bath, Miss Levy noticed that he coughed frequently, especially when he moved from one position to another. She also noticed that he wasn't spitting up any sputum and that his lips and nails were slightly blue. Miss Levy reported this to her team leader. A doctor came and checked Mr. Snyder's heart and lungs. He ordered rest and medications. Mr. Snyder was experiencing congestive heart failure.

SMELLING

The sense of smell is as important as hearing and seeing, although it is often taken for granted. When we eat, the senses of seeing, tasting, and smelling give us our impressions of the different kinds of food. Smell can be an important aid in observing your patients.

While helping Mrs. Grant with her bath, Miss Fitzgerald noticed that she was not as talkative as usual. In fact, she fell asleep twice. While dozing, she breathed heavily and her breath smelled like sweet ripe fruit. Miss Fitzgerald reported all this to the nurse. Because of her observations, Mrs. Grant, who was a diabetic, was found to be going into a diabetic coma and was treated in time.

TOUCHING

Many observations can be made by touching, which enables the nursing assistant to determine whether the patient's skin is hot or cold, wet or dry, firm or flabby, strong or weak, smooth or coarse. Many people are afraid to touch. In our North American culture people do not touch casually very much, but nursing assistants will find that touching is one of their most valuable observation tools.

One evening, as Miss Jones was giving Mr. Fernandez a backrub, she noticed that he felt hot. She took his temperature—it was 103°. She reported this immediately. The charge nurse had been in and seen Mr. Fernandez only 15 minutes before to give him medication, but she had not touched him, and had not discovered the problem. As a result of Miss Jones's action, Mr. Fernandez, who had leukemia, was treated immediately. Otherwise, he would have run a fever all night and become seriously dehydrated and ill.

USING ALL YOUR SENSES FOR ACCURATE OBSERVATION

You need to use all your senses in order to observe accurately and fully. You need to look and perceive, listen, smell, and touch in order to get the whole message or picture.

Observe your patients every day. Some observations you make are included on the care plan. These include taking and recording temperature and pulse, and recording stools and fluid intake and output. Every day, you should check your patients systematically, from head to toe. You should ask yourself the following questions:

- How does this person normally behave?
- How does he usually look?
- What does he usually do?
- How does he usually speak?
- What does he talk about?

You should also observe what your patients can do for themselves. Even if it takes more patience on your part, you should encourage them to do as much as they can. Write down what your patients can do, and tell other staff members. Too many people make judgments about what their patients can do without carefully observing and talking with them.

Observing for Changes

You should also watch for changes in your patients. Anything about them that seems different should be reported. Changes in voice or speech, eyes, size of pupils, manner of walking, appetite, urine or stool, behavior, or mental status should all be reported. Investigate the circumstances of the change carefully. A person may seem confused because he has misplaced his glasses or some other possession. You can easily correct this. Maybe he is confused because he is constipated or because he is going into heart failure.

Some other important observations that should be reported and recorded are:

Pain	Rash
Swelling	Dizziness, feeling faint
Numbness	Nausea, vomiting
Cough	Abdominal swelling
Discoloration of skin, eyes	Hiccoughs
Breaks in the skin	Belching
(especially over bony	Passing flatus
prominences and on	Drainage (from eyes,
the feet)	ears, mouth, rectum,
Chills	or wounds)
Itching	Excessive perspiration

Any of the above could be an indication of some disease process or some harmful change in the body that could be helped or prevented by treatment.

You should be observing your patients throughout your entire shift. Whether you are admitting a new resident or helping patients bathe, shower, dress, walk, exercise, or socialize, observe them constantly. Be alert while giving an enema, applying a hot or cold pack, emptying a commode or bedpan, assisting with eating, making a bed or talking with a patient. You should be continuously observing your patients' surroundings for safety hazards, adequate drinking water, misplaced possessions, and so on.

Observations on Evening and Night Shifts

Observations should also take place throughout the evening and night shifts. The nursing assistant who works at night must make a special effort to use every contact with his or her patients to its fullest extent. Because these contact times are so limited, he or she must develop good observation techniques. Talk to patients who are awake. Be sure there is enough light for you to see them and for them to see you. Listen carefully, and touch an arm or a hand. Excessive perspiration could be a sign of too many bed covers, fever, or an insulin reaction in a diabetic. Sometimes the only way this sign can be discovered at night is by touch. Talk to patients who seem confused. Try to find out why this is happening, and reorient them by telling them who you are and where they are. Record behavior changes carefully. Often these may occur only at night. Your recorded and reported observations are the only means by which nurses and doctors can know about them.

REPORTING OBSERVATIONS

All observations must be reported. In most institutions these would be reported to the team leader or the charge nurse. Even if you have made no special observation, you should report to this person about one hour before the end of your shift. Report what happened to your patients during the shift. It is your responsibility to find out who to report to during your shift.

Sometimes you may feel that the person to whom you give the report does not think your observation is important. No observation is stupid. With experience, you will discover which observations are the most important. However, if you feel something needs further investigation, repeat yourself and ask again if the nurse will come and look at the patient. Sometimes the nurse may be trying to handle more than one problem or to listen to more than one person at a time.

A good time to emphasize observations you have made is during the team conference when there is discussion about your patient. The purpose of these conferences is to get to understand each patient and his problems better, and to make the best plan of care possible for him. Without your observations, this plan may not be complete.

RECORDING OBSERVATIONS

You must record as well as report all observations. Some facilities have checklists or assessment sheets on which nursing assistants can check how the patient is progressing in his eating, dressing, washing, etc. Some facilities have clip boards at the desk on which notes can be written. In some nursing homes, nursing assistants write their observations on the nurses' notes or the patients' charts.

When you write down your observations, write what your senses tell you. Do not write your opinion.

CORRECT: *Bright red spot, 6 in. wide, on sheet.*
                                                   – D. Kerr
INCORRECT: *Much blood on sheet. – D. Kerr*

CORRECT: *Sitting alone in room all day. Says does not want to talk. Crying at times.*
INCORRECT: *Depressed. – D. Kerr*   *– D. Kerr*

CORRECT: *Says, "No one cares about me." – D. Kerr*
INCORRECT: *Feels alone and depressed. – D. Kerr*

CORRECT: *Says, "This is one of my best days in weeks." – D. Kerr*
INCORRECT: *Good day. – D. Kerr*

Write about changes. If the patient was able to wash more or less of himself than usual, or ate more or less than usual, record this.

CORRECT: *5/10/19–. 3 p.m. Washed self. Sat in living room most of day. Assisted to walk in hall every two hours. – D. Kerr*
INCORRECT: *Bath. Routine day. – D. Kerr*

Write what you did to prevent possible problems. Write about who you turned, positioned, exercised and so on, and when you did these things.

Sharpening Your Observations

You need to practice your observation skills every day. Try to be more aware of what you see, hear, smell, and touch. Some nursing assistants carry checklists around with them to remind them what to look for.

One way of sharpening your observation skills is to play a mental game with yourself. At the beginning of the shift, choose one part of the body that you are going to observe very carefully on each of your patients. If, for example, you choose "hands," what can you observe by looking at and touching people's hands? There are the colors of hands and nails, thinness, size of knuckles, amount of stiffening of the joints, dryness of skin, temperature, evidence of pain on movement, strength of grasp, shakiness or steadiness, broken areas on skin, condition of nails (cracked, very short, very long, thick, dirty, manicured), and how each person uses his hands to express himself. You can tell much about people just by observing their hands. If you look carefully at different parts of the body, you will soon become a much more skillful observer.

SUMMARY

Observation makes the difference between a good and an excellent nursing assistant. The nursing assistant who is able to do the tasks of her job well is important to patients and team. But the nursing assistant who observes each individual patient and attempts to determine his or her status each day is even more important.

Mr. Canter complained to Mrs. Owalski that he felt as if he had to go to the bathroom to urinate. Mrs. Owalski knew something was wrong because Mr. Canter had a catheter tube in his bladder. All the urine was supposed to flow automatically out of the tube and into a bag beside his bed. She put her hand where his hand was—on his lower abdomen. It felt very hard. She looked at the tubing and collection bag. Both were empty. Then she saw that Mr. Canter was lying on the tubing, which was kinked. He had been lying on it for about two hours. She reported this immediately, and also unkinked the tube. Mr. Canter became comfortable again.

DISCUSSION QUESTIONS

1.   How well do you observe your patients?

2.   How many meaningful observations could you make from looking at your patients' feet? faces? backs?

3.   How can incomplete observation interfere with patient care?

4.   What are the possible differences between these two observations: "Patient depressed." "Patient says, 'I am unhappy.' "?

5.   Make a checklist of observations that should be made of your patients' rooms.

6.   Make a checklist of observations that need to be made daily to keep you aware of your patients' abilities to do or not do things for themselves.

7

The Nursing Home: A Humane Environment

All behavior, no matter how ridiculous it may seem, has some meaning. It has a need-meeting purpose. We all use certain behaviors to meet needs in our lives. These behaviors help us to maintain a certain level of mental and physical comfort.

We learn much of our behavior as we are growing up. We learn how we should behave in order to fit in at certain places and with certain people (in church, at a football game, on a date, at a town meeting). We learn the appropriate behavior for the roles we fill during life—roles such as student, mother, father, doctor, nursing assistant, nurse, and even patient.

Much of our behavior helps us and others to define who we are and what we are. Our behavior and our patients' behavior set the tone of the nursing home.

FEELINGS ABOUT NURSING HOMES

Many people have negative feelings about entering nursing homes as guests or as patients or even as employees. They have heard stories about patients who quickly changed for the worse after entering a nursing home. To most people, a nursing home means an institution, not a "home."

Studies have been done to find out how elderly people are affected by moving from their homes to nursing homes. It has been found that this often causes confusion and withdrawal. Moving to a nursing home usually involves many losses, such as the loss of a home, friends, and possessions. The patient does not usually expect to gain new friends or new possessions in the nursing home. He has a dread of what the future holds.

The older person does not know how to act in the role of a chronically ill patient in a nursing home.[1] The acutely ill person in a hospital knows that he must follow the doctor's and nurse's orders, and that he will go home when he is better. The chronically ill older person in a nursing home does not know what to expect. He does not know how to act. He does not know whether he will go home. Will he be allowed to be sick and get help on the days when he is not feeling well? And will he be able to do what he wants on other days when he feels fine?

Some people who work in nursing homes also seem to be confused about their roles and their patients' roles. They may make the residents of nursing homes more dependent by thinking of themselves as nursing the sick and dying. Instead, they should think of themselves as helpers whose role is to teach older people how to compensate for their losses.

It is the job of everyone in a long-term care facility to set a positive tone that will make entering and living in an "institution" easier. Colorful walls and curtains help create this kind of an environment, but they are not enough. It is the behavior of the people who work in the nursing home that makes the difference. Residents sense how well or badly workers get along with one another and with other patients. Just as members of the staff judge patients, so patients judge staff by their behavior.

A staff that can work together and help one another usually does a good job of helping patients. When members of the staff do not get along, the solution is to have a face-to-face discussion about their problems. Usually there is someone in the facility who is a good group leader. Some nursing homes bring in outside consultants specially trained to help people learn to understand their jobs and one another through group discussion. The nursing home staff members should give residents the impression that they are working together. They should not talk about other staff members or discuss staff problems with residents.

IMPORTANCE OF THE FIRST IMPRESSION

The first impression received by patients entering nursing homes is extremely important. Patients should be greeted by someone who is friendly and willing to give them helpful information about their new residence. This person should help them become oriented to their rooms and to what belongs to them, such as their bedside stand, bureau, bathroom, and so on.

At the beginning, every new resident should meet one person who will see him repeatedly throughout the first weeks. This person could be a nursing assistant or nurse, or even a nonnursing person who visits the patient once a day to find out how he is doing and what he needs.

Often patients are very concerned over the few possessions they have left. They are distressed when their things are taken or misplaced. They need someone whom they feel is on their side, who will stand up for their rights, and who will listen to their complaints. They need to establish a relationship with a person whom they feel they can trust and call upon in times of distress.

The first impression of the nursing home received by the family and friends of new residents is also important. They should be greeted politely and respectfully. If they wish to give information about the patient's habits and way of life, the nursing assistant should listen carefully and report the information to the charge nurse.

THE PATIENT'S FAMILY

Sometimes staff members blame family members for the problems of elderly patients. The family's behavior toward the patient must be considered in terms of a lifetime of interaction between patient and family. Maybe they have fought all of their lives. Maybe they dislike one another. Maybe the patient's children feel guilty about putting their parent in a nursing home. It is difficult to see one's parents as weak and dependent instead of strong. Sometimes a social worker can help family members and residents understand and cope with their feelings.

HELPING THE PATIENT ADJUST EMOTIONALLY

The new resident of a nursing home should not be expected to adjust to his or her situation for weeks and sometimes months. During a resident's first few weeks in a home, his behavior may change so much that his family may say he is not himself. His new behavior may be the only way he has of coping with a situation where he feels he has lost control. In a pleasant and positive environment, this change in behavior will probably be temporary.

The things that affect the behavior of each of us also affect the behavior of older people. These include not only our environment, our present situation, our needs, and our experiences, but also our feelings.

Our feelings affect our behavior. Because of the many sudden losses and changes in elderly patients' lives, they experience many feelings. A person of any age who had such losses and changes would feel the same way. But older people may have less ability to cope with their feelings.

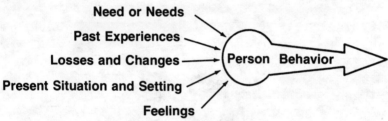

Need or Needs

Past Experiences

Losses and Changes ──→ **Person Behavior**

Present Situation and Setting

Feelings

A person's behavior is influenced by many things.

Guilt

Older people often feel guilty. Old age is a time of thinking back on the past and looking for a meaning to one's life. If wrongs were done or grudges held, older people may try to make up for this. They may become more religious or want to talk about their "sins."[2] It is important to allow patients to talk about what they feel they've done in the past. They can then feel more comfortable.

Loneliness

Older people often feel lonely. They often feel abandoned and deserted by their friends and families and their own bodies. When they lose the feeling that they can control their lives, they feel helpless and useless.

Grief

Older people often feel grief over the loss of a loved one or object. Such a loss may cause them to become immobilized or slowed down for as long as six to twelve months. They may

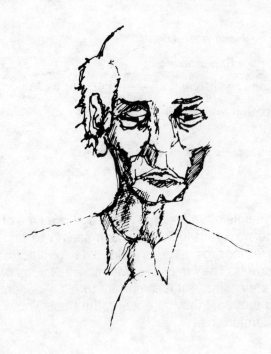

become very irritable and confused and be unable to eat or sleep. They may become seriously depressed and physically or mentally ill. Older people may also grieve for no apparent cause. They may be anticipating their own deaths or the deaths of others.[3] Grieving people should be encouraged to talk about and show their feelings. They should be able to talk about death. They should not be isolated.

Anxiety

Older people are often anxious. Anxiety is a dread of, or uneasy feeling about, the unknown future. It causes many physical signs, among them sweaty hands, frequent urination, pinpoint pupils, constipation. Any new experience may cause older people anxiety. They need a lot of support, explanation, and honest praise for everything they attempt. They may express anxiety in many ways. Some may use selective hearing[4]—"He only hears what he wants to hear." Some may call the nursing assistant frequently for no apparent reason. Some may be suspicious of everyone and accuse people of taking their possessions. These people need someone they can trust who will come when they call or will find their misplaced items.

Rage

Older people often feel a sense of rage at all the uncontrollable things that are happening to them,[5] and at being neglected and humiliated in many little ways. Rage may be expressed by shouting and hitting or by holding in one's feelings. Sometimes the things that have caused the rage can be changed or ironed out by the nursing assistant.

Nursing assistants should let their patients express their feelings, even hostile ones. They should listen carefully and try to understand what the person is saying or why he is doing something. They should try to think of a patient's less acceptable behavior as a call for help, a call to "look, listen, and understand me." Almost all such pleas for help can be responded to in some positive way that will make the patient's life a little better or prevent it from becoming worse.

Feelings and Behavior

People react differently to their feelings. Some try to discover the reason for them and do something about them. Some try to deny that their feelings exist, while others blame everyone else or the world situation for the way they feel. Some look to the past and blame deceased relatives, and others become very busy, or very dependent, or very blind, or very deaf. By acting in these ways they are able to keep in control of themselves and accept themselves from day to day.

THE DEPRESSED PATIENT

The most prevalent emotional illness of older people is depression. This is an illness that is curable. But, if it is not cured or helped, it could lead to suicide. In fact, the highest successful suicide rate occurs among white men in their eighties.

Depression is thought to be a person's reaction to a loss, whether it is a real or imaginary loss. The signs and symptoms of depression vary widely from patient to patient and include insomnia, drowsiness, loss of appetite, gain of appetite, loss of interest, a general slowing down, or continuous moving and doing.

Nursing assistants should watch for changes in their patients' usual behavior and report these to their charge nurses. Usually a doctor, preferably a psychiatrist, will see the patient, and medications will be ordered. After the medications have been taken, it is very important to observe and report the patient's behavior so that it can be decided whether the medications have helped.

Nursing assistants can be extremely helpful to persons who are depressed. Usually these patients feel helpless, hopeless, unwanted, and unloved. They need someone who will listen to them and help them take a realistic look at themselves. They usually underrate themselves. They cannot and should not be humored or cajoled out of their feelings. They should be taken very seriously, no matter how inconsequential their problems seem.

Because the signs and symptoms of depression vary so much, it often goes undiagnosed in the elderly population. Older people who exhibit rapid changes of behavior are often called "flaky" or "senile" when, in fact, they are seriously depressed.

THE PATIENT WITH CHRONIC ORGANIC BRAIN SYNDROME

Chronic organic brain syndrome (sometimes called senility) is a mental disorder of older people caused by the death of many vital brain cells. Some of the signs of this disorder include disorientation, memory loss, poor judgment, frequent mood changes such as sudden anger for no apparent reason, and an increasing inability to take care of one's own needs.

Older people with true chronic organic brain syndrome may have permanent behavior changes. Many older people, however, may have some of the symptoms of this syndrome temporarily. The memory loss, mood swings, and confusion may be caused by any one of the following: anxiety, fear, grief, depression, fever, infection, malnutrition, dehydration, constipation, drug reactions, disease, decreased capacity to see or hear, transfer to a nursing home or to a new room in a nursing home, and lack of human contact and mental stimulation.

Don't expect that all of the patients who come to nursing homes with a diagnosis of senility or chronic organic brain syndrome will act in the same way. Each person is an individual and will behave differently. Observe each carefully and describe, record, and report their behaviors. Most of these people can benefit from more than custodial care. By repetition and reorientation, many can be retaught the activities of daily living and can function on a higher level. Because symptoms similar to those of chronic organic brain syndrome may be caused by any of the factors mentioned above, it is not fair to form opinions about elderly patients until they have been in the institution for a while and are known as individuals.

THE CONFUSED PATIENT

Confusion is a term used by nurses and nursing assistants to describe behavior and speech that seems disorganized or "out of touch with reality." When you call a patient confused, describe exactly what he did or said that made you believe this was so. When your patient seems confused, listen to what he or she is saying. Try to make sense of it. Do not laugh. Some older people confuse words. They may say "mother" when they mean "daughter," but they know what they mean. Many forget the day or date because their days and weeks are all so much alike.

Some patients have hallucinations. This means they see people or objects that do not exist. If your patient is having hallucinations, make it clear to him that what may seem real for him is not real for you. When Mrs. Donovan thinks she sees a mouse on the floor, do not say to her, "It's not there." Instead, say, "I don't see it." Don't make the person feel that he is lying or silly, but indicate that there is a difference between what you see and what he sees, and that this is a problem. Some patients have "patchy" confusion. They are confused sometimes and not at other times. If you play along with their hallucinations, they may realize, during a more lucid time, that this is what you were doing. Then they will lose trust in you and feel that you are always belittling or humoring them.

Try to keep nursing home residents in contact with what is real as much as possible. Have large numbered calendars in all the rooms. These can be obtained from stationers or banks. Circle the date each day. The clocks on the walls should have large faces. Remind your patients what time it is and show them the clock. At the beginning of each shift, remind them when meals will be served. Do this again before each meal. This gives some structure to the day. When you greet your patients each morning, remind them what day and date it is, and where they are. Call them by their proper name or the name by which they wish to be called. "Good morning, Mr. Babcock. It's a warm, sunny Tuesday in April, April 18, 19__. I'm Mrs. Delgado, your nursing assistant at Dale Nursing Home." Some institutions have this kind of information spoken over the paging system each morning. Meals can also be announced in this way. Some homes have information about the date and the weather and meals written on "orientation" bulletin boards. Residents are reminded to look at these each day.

When speaking to confused patients, use simple statements and questions. Repeat everything as often as necessary. Never speak to other people about these patients or about their confusion in their presence. You can't assume that they will not understand you.

Touching is a very important part of reorientation. People respond to messages of warmth and friendliness given through touch.

A regularly scheduled group discussion led by a nursing assistant specially trained in reorientation and remotivation therapy[6] can be very helpful to confused and withdrawn patients. This kind of group work has helped patients become orientated and more independent. It has stimulated them to think and speak, and has increased their self-esteem. The subjects of discussion in these groups are things that people are involved with in their day-to-day lives, such as food, events, holidays, familiar objects, and nature.

THE HOSTILE PATIENT

When you have a patient who is verbally abusive, listen to what he is saying. Don't try to talk him out of his feelings. Try to find a reason for the behavior. If something in the environment is bothering him, attempt to change it if that is possible. Sometimes the wrong food or a lack of privacy may be the "last straw" in a number of annoying incidents. Be consistent and trustworthy in your behavior toward him. Any inconsistency may be taken as a slight.

Restraints should be used only when the patient's safety or that of other patients is seriously in question. They should not be used as a substitute for the presence of a nurse or nursing assistant. The patient who must be restrained should ordinarily not be isolated. It would usually be better to bring him to a central area where he can see other people and be greeted by nurses and other patients. For some, however, this might be too stimulating and cause further confusion, and for some it might be too humiliating.

The patient who is restrained feels humiliated and less like a person. He feels he has lost control over his environment. Any restraint should be removed every two hours and the patient should be examined and observed for possible ill effects.

The staff that works with a patient who is abusive and combative needs continual support. They need to get together on a regular basis and talk about their feelings (good and bad) toward the patient. They need to talk about and plan the kind of approach they will all consistently use with him.

STAFF BEHAVIOR AFFECTS PATIENTS' BEHAVIOR

Reward is a means of changing people's behaviors. In some institutions residents are given money, or tokens that can be used for money, if they perform certain tasks, such as mopping the floor, emptying wastebaskets, and so on. This encourages them to keep their ward clean and do useful work.

Generally, people feel good about themselves and repeat

what they are doing when they are rewarded for doing it. Sometimes, especially with a patient who exhibits uncontrollable or unconventional behavior, the nursing team may plan to reward certain behavior in order to discourage other behavior. This is a type of behavior modification therapy.[7]

Rewards do not need to be money or possessions. They can also be a smile or warm, affectionate praise. For example, the nursing staff and doctor in one nursing home planned an approach for a patient who insisted on eating with his hands. They decided to put a spoon in his hand each time any of them walked in his room and found him eating with his hands. If he ate with the spoon, they would smile and praise him warmly. If he did not, they would leave the room. Slowly, he began to eat with a spoon.

Using rewards to change behavior should only be done when this is a planned part of nursing care and is carried out by the entire team. The reward should be given every time the desired behavior appears. If this does not happen, the patient could become confused.

You should be aware of how your behavior affects your patients—whether it is hurting or helping them. Sometimes you may not realize that you are encouraging undesirable behavior in the person you are trying to help.

Mrs. Flaubert is an 80-year-old woman who becomes so extremely anxious at night that she very frequently pushes the call button. When the nursing assistant asks what she wants, she says she doesn't know. As a result, she has been getting fewer answers to her calls. But when she wets the bed and calls about that, the nursing assistant stays with her, washes her, and changes her bed.

Mrs. Flaubert is frightened of being alone. She has found that wetting the bed keeps someone in the room with her. The nursing assistant is encouraging Mrs. Flaubert to wet the bed by not spending enough time with her. If she had stayed with Mrs. Flaubert and talked with her a little longer the first time she was called, she probably would have discovered that Mrs. Flaubert was afraid of being alone at night. Then the nursing assistant might have made more of an effort to help her patient become comfortable and relaxed. She might have offered her a warm drink, help to the bathroom, a backrub, and the reassurance that she would come if called. Possibly Mrs. Flaubert would then have fallen asleep at the beginning of the night and remained so all night long.

SUMMARY

The behaviors of your patients give you some clues to what they are feeling and what they need. But behavior is to the total person as the tip of the iceberg is to what lies below. It can be deceiving. It may give you clues you cannot understand. In order to understand these clues, you need to know your patients well. Talk with them and listen to them. By being aware of the influences, including yourself, on your patients' behaviors, and by trying to make these influences positive, you can help create a humane environment in your nursing facility.

REFERENCES

[1]Katherine M. Ness, "The Sick Role of the Elderly," from *Psycho-Social Nursing Care of the Aged,* Ed. by Irene Mortenson Burnside (New York: McGraw-Hill Book Company, 1973), pp. 55-69.

[2]Robert N. Butler, and Myrna I. Lewis, *Aging and Mental Health* (St. Louis: The C.V. Mosby Company, 1973), p. 37.

3Ibid., p. 37.
4Ibid., p. 39.
5Ibid., p. 39.
6If you are interested in this type of training, contact your State Association of Certified Remotivation. You could also write for information to the National Remotivation Training Center, Philadelphia State Hospital, Philadelphia, Pennsylvania.
7Michael D. LeBow, *Behavior Modification, A Significant Method in Nursing Practice* (Englewood Cliffs, New Jersey: Prentice-Hall, Inc., 1973), pp. 69-96.

DISCUSSION QUESTIONS

1. What information do you need to know about your patients in order to understand their behavior better?

2. Think of ways in which your patients have expressed feelings of guilt, grief, anxiety, and rage.

3. Can you think of a patient whose behavior you misinterpreted?

4. What do you consider inappropriate behavior for people who live in long-term care facilities? Why?

5. Would you like to be a resident in the nursing home or long-term care facility in which you work? Why? Why not?

6. What kinds of changes would make your facility a more pleasant place to live and work in? How can these changes be made? Is there anything *you* can do to make it more pleasant?

8

Role-Plays

A NOTE ON ROLE-PLAYING

Role-playing is a way of learning how to handle real life situations in a classroom or group setting. It helps you gain insight into how another person sees his world. It gives you a chance to practice certain skills, such as how to talk with a patient, how to solve a particular problem, or how to do a particular procedure.

Most role-plays are quite structured. This means that you are given information from which you must act a part. You are expected to act like the person whom you are supposed to be, rather than acting like yourself. Other role-plays may be more spontaneous. For example, when you are discussing a problem at a conference, your group leader might say, "You be Mr. Ching and I'll be the nurse. Let's talk about it."

Those who are observing the role-play have just as much responsibility as those who are acting in it. The observers should watch how each actor's behavior affects the other actors, and what is being said and done. When the group leader asks, "What happened?" give your impression of the role-play and what you think it meant.

103

The role-play should last no longer than five minutes. It should take place where everyone in the group who is not acting can see and hear what is happening. This method works best in a group in which people know one another and are willing to join in.

ROLE-PLAY ONE

Theme: Physical and mental activity is important for maintenance of health.

Characters:

> *NURSING ASSISTANT PAMELA GRAY.* Mr. Papadapoulos sits in his chair from morning to night. His only activity is getting up to go to the bathroom three or four times a day. His meals are served to him in his room. You are concerned about this lack of activity, and want to talk with him about it.

> *MR. PAPADAPOULOS:* You sit in your chair all day. No one visits you. You have few interests any more.

ROLE-PLAY TWO

Theme: Communication between staff members provides useful information for nursing care.

Characters:

MR. POLANSKI: You are an 84-year-old widower who has been living in this facility for the past six months. Formerly, you were a carpenter. You are a devout Catholic and have attended the chapel service every day since you arrived. But the past two mornings, when the nursing assistant asked if you were going to get ready to go to chapel, you became angry and yelled, "Get out and leave me alone. You don't understand!"

NURSE MARIA DIAZ: You are sitting with two nursing assistants during a coffee break, discussing this problem. You have only worked in this facility for a month.   Mr. Polanski has not been a problem to you in the past, but now you are bothered by his yelling because it upsets the other patients. This, in turn, disturbs the director of nursing. Yesterday you tried to give Mr. Polanski a tranquilizer to control his behavior, but he refused to let you.

NURSING ASSISTANT JOAN McGREGGOR: You have been working as a nursing assistant here for two years. You have always liked Mr. Polanski. You realize that he is a man who likes things in order and on schedule. You feel that possibly Mrs. Jones, who has been taking care of him for the last two days, has been rushing him. You want to tell her this, but you don't know how to do this without offending her.

NURSING ASSISTANT NANCY JONES: You have been working here for three years. You feel tired and overworked. Mr. Polanski's yelling has been annoying you and you feel he is just being stubborn. You feel that ignoring this behavior would be the best way to stop it. You think that if he gets worse, he should be restrained. There are too many other patients who need care.

ROLE-PLAY THREE

Theme: Assessment of each older person's needs is a necessary part of caring.

Characters:

NURSING ASSISTANT PAT HERADA: You just saw Alice Bixby, nursing assistant, put Mrs. Vanderveer on a bedpan and then "diaper" her. You are concerned because you know that Mrs. Vanderveer has been on a bladder training program for the last week. She is to be put on a commode on arising in the morning, before and after each meal, and before going to bed at night. This is hard work, but already you have seen results.

Mrs. Vanderveer hasn't been incontinent for two days. You signal Miss Bixby to step out into the hall with you.

NURSING ASSISTANT ALICE BIXBY: You have not taken care of this patient for two weeks. Then she was incontinent two or three times a day, and used the bedpan at other times. After you finished putting Mrs. Vanderveer on the bedpan just now, you "diapered" her because it seemed the best way to keep her from wetting the bed. There isn't much linen left.

ROLE-PLAY FOUR

Theme: Reporting observations is a nursing assistant's responsibility.

Characters:

NURSING ASSISTANT JAN CHOW: While washing Mrs. Amata's feet, you notice that her right great toe is a bluish color. She complains about pain in it. When you examine the toe closely, you see a half-inch cut on it. But yesterday there was no cut or bluish color on the toe or you would have noticed it. You decide to report this to a nurse.

CHARGE NURSE JEROME LEVY: You are a charge nurse preparing a pain medication for a patient who has been asking for it for over half an hour. And *now* Miss Chow wants to talk to you! You feel hurried.

ROLE-PLAY FIVE

Theme: Behavior is a response to unmet needs.

Characters:

> *MR. ALBERT SAROYAN:* You are a 74-year-old resident who suffered a stroke three years ago. As a result, you must move about in a wheel chair. You have been lonely since your last roommate was transferred to another nursing home. You have been looking forward to a new roommate, who has just arrived.

> *MR. LARS LARSEN:* You are 80 years old. You have just been transferred from another nursing home to this one because of finances. You were comfortable in the other place. You don't understand why you had to move. You don't want to talk to anyone. You are having trouble finding all your things in your suitcase, and you don't know where the bathroom is! You don't like being called "gramps" by the nursing assistant. Anyone that young should call you Mr. Larsen. You feel like crying.

> *NURSING ASSISTANT CARMEN MENDOZA:* You bring in Mr. Larsen, who seems irritable. You introduce him to his roommate, Mr. Saroyan. You think Mr. Larsen will feel more comfortable if you call him "gramps," so you do this. You tell him where his dresser and closet are.

ROLE-PLAY SIX (This is a less structured role-play.)

Theme: Role-playing helps nursing assistants understand their patients' feelings.

Characters:

> *NURSING ASSISTANT:* You are to feed the patient.

> *PATIENT:* You are to be fed. Act like a particular patient in your facility with whom a feeding problem has arisen lately.

Change roles and try again.

9

Case Studies

CASE STUDY ONE

Mr. Ledbetter is a 60-year-old ex-high school history teacher who has had a stroke. He cannot speak except for some repetitive speech and profanity. He has lost control of his bladder. He is right-handed and his right side is paralyzed. His left arm and hand are weak. He can barely lift a full coffee cup without spilling it.

Mr. Ledbetter can feed himself if he is placed in a chair. This is rarely done because he is such a big, heavy man. Besides, he makes such a mess when he feeds himself. He grabs at the food in front of him and stuffs it in his mouth. The right side of his face sags. Without realizing it, he soon collects a pocket of food between his cheek and teeth on the right side. When he drinks, he drools and spills.

Mr. Ledbetter's wife visits him, but she feels she cannot help him. She is embarrassed by his profanity. Some nursing assistants are afraid of him because he "reminds them of pictures of the devil" with his black bushy eyebrows and leering facial expression.

At morning report, the night nurse says that Mr. Ledbetter was incontinent five times during the night. She changed the linen each time, but it seemed almost futile to try to keep the bed dry. She says he needs to be fed.

What if Mr. Ledbetter were your patient?

The ideas for this case study were taken from Mary Opal Wolanin, "They Called the Patient Repulsive," *American Journal of Nursing* 64:73-75.

DISCUSSION QUESTIONS

1. What needs must you, the nursing assistant, help Mr. Ledbetter meet?

2. What are Mr. Ledbetter's remaining strengths? How can they be used to help make up for his weaknesses?

3. In what nonverbal ways might Mr. Ledbetter communicate with you? What verbal ways?

4. What self-help devices and arrangements within Mr. Ledbetter's room could be used to help him help himself?

5. Review transfer procedures that might be used to help Mr. Ledbetter move from bed to chair.

6. How might the nursing assistants who fear Mr. Ledbetter be helped to know him better and understand his problems?

7. How might Mr. Ledbetter's incontinence be managed?

8. How do you think Mr. Ledbetter feels?

CASE STUDY TWO

Mr. Minolka is 89 years old and has been living in the nursing home for ten years. He originally came with his wife, who was quite ill. She died a little less than a year ago.

Mr. Minolka used to spend his time carving wooden spoons and bowls or reading, but for the last six weeks he has been sitting in a chair in his room with his head bowed. He eats much less than he used to. Woodworking and reading have been difficult lately because of changes in his vision. He can see forms and shadows, but must be very close to a person or object to distinguish features. When the nursing assistant encourages him to wear his glasses, he says "they don't work."

Sometimes Mr. Minolka seems confused. He can't remember where he is and calls for his wife. Some of the nursing staff say he is getting "senile."

DISCUSSION QUESTIONS

1. How can you help a person with visual loss maintain his independence and interest? How could you help Mr. Minolka know who you are, where you are, and what you are doing?

2. How would you describe Mr. Minolka's behavior? Write your observations.

3. What do you think Mr. Minolka is feeling? Why do you think he acts as he does? What losses has he experienced in the last year?

4. What does senile mean? How can you help a confused person remain oriented? What are some reasons why an elder living in a nursing home might become confused?

CASE STUDY THREE

Mrs. Harris is a 76-year-old widow. She has been a resident of the nursing home for five years.

Because of severe rheumatoid arthritis, Mrs. Harris cannot move well. Her joints are stiff and painful. She can hardly raise her hands to her face because of shoulder and elbow contractures. She has difficulty holding anything in her hands, including silverware, because of severe contractures of her fingers.

Mrs. Harris can bear weight on her feet long enough to be helped to a chair, but it causes her pain. Two people need to help her do this. She can sit in her chair for about two hours without pain. It is at this time that she eats lunch and reads mystery stories or the Bible.

Mrs. Harris eats small amounts of food. She has become thinner, but not underweight. She eats best when sitting up. She has had choking spells when lying down and fears future ones. Because her gums have shrunk and her dentures no longer fit, she has to eat ground and pureed foods.

When in bed, Mrs. Harris can assist the nurse who turns her from side to side, but this gives her a great deal of pain. She uses the bedpan with help. She can only reach her signal light when it is placed on her chest. Her voice is a whisper. She is slightly hard of hearing, has a hearing aid, but will not wear it because it "doesn't fit," she says.

Mrs. Harris has an open pressure area about the size of a dime on the back of her head. She has a draining wound on her sacrum. This is due to pressure and a bone infection. It is covered with a dressing which often becomes soiled when she uses the bedpan.

Mrs. Harris does not have much opportunity to talk with the staff or other residents. However, she is visited every day by her son or a friend. She goes to the son's house in a wheelchair on holidays, but this is becoming harder for her because being moved and sitting for long periods of time is painful and tiring. She is embarrassed when her grandchildren see how clumsily she handles her fork and knife when she eats.

DISCUSSION QUESTIONS

1. What needs must the nursing assistant help Mrs. Harris meet?

2. What problems interfere with Mrs. Harris' ability to help herself?

3. What are Mrs. Harris' remaining strengths? How can she use these to make her life more pleasant and comfortable?

4. What self-help devices and room arrangements could be used to help Mrs. Harris?

5. What problems have developed because Mrs. Harris has not moved or been moved properly and enough? How can these problems be kept from getting worse?

6. How are Mrs. Harris' senses impaired? What can be done to increase what she can hear and see from her bed or chair? her opportunities for taste? her opportunities to touch and be touched?

7. How does Mrs. Harris feel about her increasing dependence on others? How could you make her feel more comfortable about this?

8. How could you help Mrs. Harris read or pursue some other interest for more than two hours a day?

CASE STUDY FOUR

Mrs. Meyer is a 72-year-old woman who lived alone until she fell and broke her left hip. After two weeks in the hospital and a hip nailing, she was brought to the nursing home.

Mrs. Meyer stays in bed most of the time, although she gets up to go to the bathroom and to sit in her chair for meals. When she transfers from bed to chair, and when she is walking, she must use a walker and put very little weight on her left leg.

Mrs. Meyer weighs 195 pounds, but this doesn't bother her. She enjoys eating, especially sweets. Unfortunately, she is a diabetic and should eat only what is on her tray. She gets extra food by coaxing her son to bring in her favorite dishes and sweets.

Because of her weight, Mrs. Meyer has difficulty turning in bed and moving in and out of bed. She perspires a great deal while in bed. She has several red areas on her back, but the skin is not broken.

When the doctor last saw Mrs. Meyer, he was concerned because she was not active enough. What would you do if she were your patient?

DISCUSSION QUESTIONS

1. What complications could Mrs. Meyer develop if she remains inactive? How can these be prevented?

2. What are some of the problems that prevent Mrs. Meyer from being more active?

3. How can these problems begin to be solved?

4. How might you and other nursing assistants get Mrs. Meyer's son involved in helping her solve some of these problems?

Bibliographies

(NOTE: A general bibliography on aging, a list of books on teaching nursing assistants, and a list of texts written especially for nursing assistants will be found at the end of this chapter-by-chapter listing.)

BIBLIOGRAPHY FOR CHAPTER TWO (A Closer Look at the Aging Process)

Curtin, Sharon R. **Nobody Ever Died of Old Age.** Boston: Little Brown and Company, 1972.

Lowy, Louis. **Training Manual for Human Service Technicians Working with Older People, Part II Trainees.** Boston: United Community Services of Greater Boston, 1968.

U.S. Department of Health, Education and Welfare. **Working with Older People: A Guide to Practice.** Public Health Service Publications: Biological, Psychological and Sociological Aspects of Aging, Vol. II No. 1459. Washington, D.C.: U.S. Government Printing Office, April, 1970.

BIBLIOGRAPHY FOR CHAPTER THREE (The Needs of the Elderly)

Anonymous. **Strike Back at Stroke.** Distributed by the American Heart Association and its Affiliates.

Anonymous. **Strokes (A Guide for the Family).** New York: American Heart Association, 1965.

Anonymous. **To Your Health. . . In Your Second Fifty Years.** Chicago: National Dairy Council, 1974.

Bergstrom, Doris, and Coles, Catherine H. **Basic Positioning Procedures.** Rehabilitation Publication 701. Minneapolis: Sister Kenny Institute, 1971.

Corliss, Edith. **Facts About Hearing and Hearing Aids.** NBS Consumer Information Series 4. Washington, D.C.: U.S. Government Printing Office, 1971.

Departments of Occupational Therapy and Nursing Education. **Self-Care for the Hemiplegic.** Rehabilitation Publication 704. Minneapolis: Sister Kenny Institute, 1970.

Flaherty, Patricia Toohey, and Jurkovich, Sandra J. **Transfers for Patients with Acute and Chronic Conditions.** Rehabilitation Publication 702. Minneapolis: Sister Kenny Institute, 1970.

Glorig, Aram, Ed. "Getting Through: A Guide to Better Understanding of the Hard of Hearing." Phonograph Record. Chicago, Illinois: Zenith Radio Corporation, 1971.

Gordon, Edward E. **Do It Yourself Again, Self-Help Devices for the Stroke Patient.** New York: American Heart Association, 1965.

Mahoney, Florence I. and Barthel, Dorothea W. **Up and Around, A Booklet to Aid the Stroke Patient in Activities of Daily Living.** The American Heart Association and its Affiliates. n.d.

Merritt, Mabel C. **Dance Therapy Program for Nursing Homes.** Boston: Department of Education and Social Concern, Unitarian Universalist Association, 1971.

Miller, Marian E. and Sachs, Marvin L. **About Bedsores, What You Need to Know to Help Prevent and Treat Them.** Philadelphia: J.B. Lippincott Company, 1974.

Schwab, Sister Marilyn. "Caring for the Aged." **American Journal of Nursing** (December 1973): 2049-2053.

Sorenson, Lois, and Ulrich, Patricia G. **Ambulation Guide for Nurses.** Rehabilitation Publication 707. Minneapolis: Sister Kenny Institute, 1974.

Stevens, Carolyn B. **Special Needs of Long-Term Patients,** Philadelphia: J.B. Lippincott Company, 1974.

Toohey, Patricia, and Larson, Corrine W. **Range of Motion Exercise: Key to Joint Mobility.** Rehabilitation Publication 703. Minneapolis: Sister Kenny Institute, 1968.

U.S. Department of Agriculture. **Food Guide for Older Folks.** Home and Garden Bulletin No. 17. Washington D.C.: U.S. Government Printing Office, August, 1974.

U.S. Department of Health, Education and Welfare. **Flexible Fashions, Clothing Tips and Ideas for the Woman with Arthritis.** Public Health Service Publication No. 1814. Washington D.C.: Government Printing Office, 1968.

U.S. Department of Health, Education and Welfare. **Working with Older People: A Guide to Practice.** Public Health Service Publications: The Aging Person: Needs and Services, Vol. III No. 1459. Washington D.C.: U.S. Government Printing Office, April, 1970.

Yates, Judith A. **Moving and Lifting Patients: Principles and Techniques.** Rehabilitation Publication 720. Minneapolis: Sister Kenny Institute, 1970.

BIBLIOGRAPHY FOR CHAPTER FOUR (Being a Helping and Caring Person)

Coombs, Arthur W., Avila, Donald L. and Purkay, W.W. **Helping Relationships: Basic Concepts for the Helping Professions.** Boston: Allyn and Bacon, Inc., 1971.

Mayeroff, Milton. **On Caring.** New York: Harper and Row, 1971.

Wolanin, Mary Opal. "They Called the Patient Repulsive." **American Journal of Nursing** 64 (June): 73-75.

BIBLIOGRAPHY FOR CHAPTER FIVE (Communication)

Cohen, Lillian Kay. **Communication Problems after a Stroke.** Rehabilitation Publication 709. Minneapolis: Sister Kenny Institute, 1971.

Kron, Thora. **Communication in Nursing.** Philadelphia: W. B. Saunders Company, 1972.
Lewis, Garland K. **Nurse-Patient Communication.** Dubuque, Iowa: Wm. C. Brown Company, 1973.
Mercer, Lianne S. and O'Connor, Patricia. **Fundamental Skills in the Nurse-Patient Relationship: A Programmed Text.** Philadelphia: W.B. Saunders Company, 1974.
O'Brien, Maureen J. **Communications and Relationships in Nursing.** St. Louis: C.V. Mosby Company, 1974.
Plachy, Roger. "I Hear You. What did you Say?" **Modern Hospital** 73 (June 1973): 111-117.

BIBLIOGRAPHY FOR CHAPTER SIX (Observation)

Byers, Virginia B. **Nursing Observation.** Dubuque, Iowa: Wm. C. Brown Company, 1973.

BIBLIOGRAPHY FOR CHAPTER SEVEN (The Nursing Home: A Human Environment)

Gibson, Allen. **The Remotivators' Guide Book.** Philadelphia: F.A. Davis Company, 1967.
Kubler-Ross, Elisabeth. **On Death and Dying.** New York: The MacMillan Company, 1969.
Preston, Tonie. "When Words Fail." **American Journal of Nursing** 73 (December 1973): 2064-2066.
U.S. Department of Health, Education, and Welfare. National Institute of Mental Health. **Mental Disorders of the Aging.** Public Health Service Publication No. 993. Washington D.C.: U.S. Government Printing Office, 1968.

GENERAL BIBLIOGRAPHIES

ON AGING AND THE AGED

deBeauvoir, Simone. **The Coming of Age.** New York: Warner Paperback Library, 1973.

Browning, Mary. **Nursing and the Aging Patient.** New York: American Journal of Nursing Company, Educational Services Division, 1974.

Butler, Robert N. and Lewis, Myrna I. **Aging and Mental Health, Positive Psychosocial Approaches.** St. Louis: The C. V. Mosby Company, 1973.

Burnside, Irene Mortenson, Ed. **Psycho-Social Nursing Care of the Aged.** New York: McGraw-Hill Book Company, 1973.

Long, Janet, M. Ed. **Caring for and Caring about Elderly People: A Guide to the Rehabilitative Approach.** Philadelphia: J.B. Lippincott Company, 1972.

TEACHING NURSING ASSISTANTS

Continuing Education Project. **Training and Continuing Education, A Handbook for Health Care Institutions.** Chicago: Hospital Research and Educational Trust, 1970.

Jaeger, Dorothea and Simmons, Leo W. **The Aged III.** New York: Appleton-Century-Crofts, 1970.

Knowles, Malcolm. **The Modern Practice of Adult Education, Andragogy versus Pedagogy.** New York: Association Press, 1970.

Lowy, Louis. **Training Manual for Human Service Technicians Working with Older Persons, Part I Trainers.** Boston: United Community Services of Greater Boston, 1968.

Maslow, Abraham. **Motivation and Personality,** New York: Harper and Brothers, Publishers.

Mayne, Marian. **A Guide to Inservice Education for Nursing Personnel in Nursing Homes.** University Extension, University of California, Los Angeles: Western Center for Continuing Education in Administration of Health Care Facilities, November 1973.

Nursing Home Trainer Program Staff, and Dickman, Irving R. **How to Plan an Inservice Education Program for your Nursing Home.** New York: Nursing Home Trainer Program, United Hospital Fund of New York, December 1972.

Scarbrough, Mrs. Dorothy, and staff. "Reality Orientation Training Program." Alabama Regional Medical Program Project. Tuscaloosa, Alabama: Veterans Administration Hospital.

Wiegand, James E. **Developing Teacher Competencies.** New Jersey: Prentice-Hall, Inc., 1971.

TEXTS WRITTEN ESPECIALLY FOR NURSING ASSISTANTS

Birchenall, Joan and Streight, Mary E. **Care of the Older Adult.** Philadelphia: J. B. Lippincott Company, 1973.

Bregman, Marcia S. **Assisting the Health Team: An Introduction for the Nurse Assistant.** St. Louis: C.V. Mosby Company, 1974.

Cherescavich, Gertrude D. **A Textbook for Nursing Assistants.** St. Louis: C.V. Mosby Company, 1973.

Gale, Charlotte B. "Walking in the Aide's Shoes." **American Journal of Nursing** (April 1973): 628-631.

Isler, Charlotte, **The Nurses Aide.** New York: Springer Publishing Company, 1973.

Reese, Dorothy Erickson. **How to be a Nurse's Aide in a Nursing Home.** Washington D.C.: The American Nursing Home Association, n.d.

Stolten, Jane H. **The Geriatric Aide.** Boston: Little, Brown and Company, 1973.

Stolten, Jane H. **The Health Aide.** Boston: Little, Brown and Company, 1972.

Audio-Visual Aids

FILM LISTINGS:

"Films on Aging," Administration on Aging catalog. For sale by the Superintendent of Documents, U.S. Government Printing Office, Washington, D.C. 20402.

"About Aging: A Film Catalog." For sale from the Publications Office, Andrus Gerontology Center, University of Southern California, University Park, Los Angeles, California.

SOME SPECIFIC FILMS:

"Perspectives on Aging."

Five filmstrips and records or cassettes.

Concept Media
1500 Adams Avenue
Costa Mesa, California 92626

"Second Chance"

About the rehabilitation of an elderly man who has had a stroke.

American Heart Association Film Library
267 W. 25th Street
New York, New York 10001
Or Your Local Chapter of the American Heart Association

"The Proud Years"

About people in their 80's and 90's who "graduate" from The Jewish Home for the Aged after being involved in a rehabilitation program.

Center for Mass Communication
Columbia University Press
440 W. 110 Street
New York, New York 10025

"Return to Reality"
"December Spring: 24 Hour Reality Orientation"
"A Time to Learn: Reality Orientation in the Nursing Home"

About the use of reality orientation techniques with confused elderly patients.

Reality Orientation Training Program
Veterans Administration Hospital
Tuscaloosa, Alabama

Index

127